American Tantra

A Modern Guide to Sacred Sex

SIENNA NEWCASTLE

iUniverse, Inc.
New York   Bloomington

iUniverse books may be ordered through booksellers or by contacting:

iUniverse
1663 Liberty Drive
Bloomington, IN 47403
www.iuniverse.com
1-800-Authors (1-800-288-4677)

ISBN: 978-1-4401-3648-1 (sc)
ISBN: 978-1-4401-3649-8 (ebook)

Printed in the United States of America

iUniverse rev. date: 04/17/2009

Dedicated to Amanda, Andy, Jennifer, and all the youth of the next generation. May these skills serve you well.

Special thanks to: Ian, Feathers, Spyder, Demian, Joe, Jason, Grim, Rose, Orbb, and Bunny for the grist in the mill. Also thanks to the Mystic Arts Gathering & Information Circle and the "Intro to Tantra Class" graduates for all the experimental guinea pigs.

Cover art by: Sienna, Rua, Spyder, and Dave

Contents

The Ego:
  "Reprogramming the Sex Instinct"
Groundwork:

  How Karezza does what it does:
  Controlling the energy of Shiva-shakti
  Why we do Karezza:
  The Kundalini path
  Time & Tantra
  What about the bad stuff?
  Exercise: Kundalini raising
  Spontaneous arousal
  Abyss or Kundalini First?
  Warning: Excessive Kundalini in one chakra will create it's
  own cure!
    So Many Men, So little Time:
  Train your brain
  Side Effects of Tantra:
  Exercise: No Fear: Meditation for Crappy Days
  Why bad things happen to good people:
  Groundwork

  Bhakti
  Gender and Tantra:
  Exercise: Making Love to Yourself:
  Exercise: Chakra Egg Meditation:
    A Party in the Heart
  American Men:
  American Women:
  What's so important about Balance?
  Orgies! Orgies everywhere!
  Bhoga:
    Learning from Bhoga:
  Groundwork:

  Introduction to Maithuna

True, Kind, Necessary
Thought, Word, Deed
Exercise: K + K
How can it possibly work?
Shortcuts:
　　A Musician's Mistake:
Picture this:
Groundwork:

Healing with the Tantric Field
Exercise: Chakra Sealing
Exercise: How to create a Tantric Field
How to play safely:
Exercise: Connecting with Nature
Resistance:
Horizontal Fields
Reverse Polarity
Negativity:
Working with untrained people:
The puppy-dog effect
　　A confidence boost:
A self-regulating field.
Orgasm Power!
Groundwork:

Puja worship history & reasons
American Pujas:
Physical side effects
Why do the puja at all?
Puja forms: White Tantra (solo)
Exercise: Shiva Puja
Shakti puja:
Double Puja--Red Tantra
Ritual Steps
　　Instant Healing (Sienna's story)
Groundwork:

Introduction:

What is American Tantra?

This book is about a spiritual practice over 5,000 years old, practiced and filtered through the most up-to-date modern civilization on this planet. American Tantra is about a religious method developed 8,000 miles away from where we are practicing, in a language that is far different from the language you are reading. American Tantra is about a union of opposites that can create peace, happiness, and prosperity in your life.

First off, what is American?

Let's start by looking at what is American anything.

American Cuisine:

Hot dogs: influenced by German sausages
Hamburgers, first made by Russians, then by Germans
Pizza, influenced by the Italians

American Entertainment:

Jazz evolved with a mixing of African, French, and Spanish culture
Rap music evolved from a mixing of tribal beats and urban experience
Hollywood is in California due to the varieties of scenery nearby

American Sports:

Baseball: adopted from the British "rounders"
Football: adopted from the British "rugby"

Basketball: created by a Canadian for New England winters

Almost everything in America came from somewhere else. Even the Native tribes that were here before the Europeans arrived were incredibly mobile. Most of them had moved onto what later became their home ranges. Without a doubt, America is a mixed bag of different cultures, influences, geography, and history, constantly changing, and surprisingly tenacious.

This is the second draft of this book, which was written during the G.W.Bush admnistration. The final edition of this book is being released within the first 100 days of the Barack Obama presidency. In the span of time it took to write and publish this book, America has changed yet again. As you read these pages, remember that not very long ago, before the time of Margaret Sanger, this information would have been illegal. The fact that it is now widely published is a testament to the changing attitudes of Americans.

So then, what is Tantra?

Tantra, in a nutshell, is a Vedic-based spiritual practice that uses physical energy, especially sexual energy, to boost human consciousness to higher states on the path to enlightenment. It's a practice 3,000 years older than the Bible, with just as many different interpretations. It's also very controversial, even in its Eastern strongholds of India and Tibet.

What I present here is not Traditional Tantra, and I will never say it is. When most Americans first hear about Tantra and the idea of Sacred Sex, the Western paradigm walls come firmly down, as they try to wrap their brains around the idea of something so crass being holy and sacred. How can something that our society teaches as "wrong" and "dirty" be a path to enlightenment? How could you possibly use sex as a way to meet Divinity?

Sex has an interesting effect on humans; we crave it, pursue it, spend time, energy, and money on it for some reason besides just procreation. (Otherwise, pregnant women would not want sex, but they do.) What's all the fuss? Orgasm. The sheer force of one orgasm can send your awareness to far-flung regions of your own imagination. Some even say that they leave their bodies if an orgasm is intense enough. Tantra gives you amazing orgasms. It's that intensity of sexual response that makes Tantra such an effective practice for spiritual enlightenment. But Tantra is about so much more than just sex.

Some people think of Tantra as large orgies of people, screwing their brains out, having orgasms with wild abandon. This is not Tantra, although in some American new age communities call it that. It isn't as simple as fueling magickal spells with orgasm, either. That's just sex magick, and while it's a lot of fun, it can't be considered entirely Tantric. Real Tantra includes a particular philosophy, certain types of meditations, and physical exercises that help you become the best 'you' that you can be, which leads to the best sex possible.

Several different "schools" and "styles" of Tantra that have been imported to America over the years. Each "school" had it's own devotees, who would interpret the Vedic scriptures individually, and then shun and disdain other "schools" as being too crass for including physical sex or too esoteric for not including it. These exclusive groups, called 'lineages,' can trace their foundations back to ancient India and the Shiva temples from thousands of years ago. While this book is not about a lineage-based system, it is still Vedic-based Tantra. I do include physical sex, but I also advocate lots and lots of training first.

Technically, Tantra is a Yoga. A "yoga" is any practice that you undertake to get closer to becoming the Divine you. Hatha yoga utilizes poses of the body to change the mindset. Yantra yoga uses images. Tantra uses all of these, which makes it a yoga of it's own. And…Tantra is the only yoga built for two.

We all have a body and a mind. The beginning exercises of Tantra aim to get you to recognize, understand, and balance these two aspects. Balancing duality between body and mind also builds up those mythic Tantric sexual abilities, like orgasm control and incredible stamina. This happens way before a student gets close to doing partnered rites.

Twilight Language:

Much of Tantric literature has been written in "twilight language," a metaphor-filled double speak that could be interpreted more than one way. For example, in some ancient texts it says to meditate until the student has obtained "release." It does not state release from what. This word can be applied to orgasmic release, stress release, release of muscular rigidity, release of the mental loops we find ourselves in, release from daily slavery, and even release from the here-and-now into some sort of trance state.

Many Tantric texts were translated from the original Sanskrit or Arabic without the benefit of the beauty of the twilight language's double-speak. Twilight language typically leaves the student asking more questions than the answers it provides. Fortunately, many scholars before us have done much of the work, and in America we can benefit from most of it.

Those mythic sexual abilities:

Tantrics have a reputation for being able to have sex for hours on end. The highest rites in paired Tantra allow for –even *require*—you to control your orgasm to make that happen. The training required for the highest Tantric rites comes in handy during any sexual activity.

To control the orgasm, you use your mind to keep control of your body while being intensely sexually stimulated. As you might imagine, this takes lots of practice. Most of this practice involves masturbating in the privacy of your own home. We call this solo work White Tantra. A typical trained Tantra practitioner has those marathon sex sessions due to all the training done masturbating. These exercises, while more fun than work, are still an important preparation for partnered Tantra.

> White Tantra:
> Tantra performed by one person

When a student gets to a certain point, he or she can begin a series of rituals for two, which don't include sex. Yet. Many students who were originally interested only in the sex drop out way before this point, so only the serious students get extended training for penetrative sexual Tantra. This aspect is called Red Tantra.

> Red Tantra:
> Tantric practice that includes combining energies of two people.

So, there is White Tantra and Red Tantra…and in American Tantra, we introduce "Blue" Tantra.

Now we can ask: What is American Tantra?

This country, once referred to as a melting pot, is now a 'tossed salad' of different cultures and backgrounds coming together. You can look at American Tantra the same way. We can't trace a single point in history where the philosophy entered this country. Many of the local Native American "Indian" religions were embracing similar concepts from the start. There are unique tribal traditions that include a type of breathing during sex that could be compared to early Tantric exercises. The concept of being here and now and in the moment was not surprising when it first fell from Eastern lips on American ears.

Some say that Tantra came to America with the Guru Craze of the 1960's. Some state a date earlier than that, during the 1920's, when Sir Arthur Avalon was publishing his first manuscripts of his travels in India. Since both of these events were more prominent in London than New York, they had only a mild impact on America. Osho, (also know as Bagwan Shri Rajneesh) made Tantra in America very popular in the 1970's and 1980's, but he and his organization fell out of favor due to political scandals that surrounded him. There truly is no one date that Tantra came to America.

In America, Tantra took root in a culture that focuses a lot on sex. Sex sells everything. We seek out sexual relationships daily. We talk about sex often. We pretend we have more than we do.

Even though lineage schools of Tantra poke fun at what they term "neo-Tantra" and "California Tantra," claiming that it is not real if it is not passed down from a lineage, Americans in the 21st century won't blindly follow anyone's beliefs without some science to back it up. We need proof, we need hands-on experience, and we need others to validate what we are experiencing.

So, this is what we get with American Tantra. We want diversity; something all-encompassing, that covers more than just the experiences of homogenous, heterosexual, white Christian European culture. We want solid results, not mythology and philosophy. We want scientific backing for our experiences, not parable and mystery. We want our chakras explained in plain English, not Sanskrit. We want hands-on exercises, not contemplations of one-hand-clapping. American Tantra does all that.

Americans want results, and we want them now. If there was ever a nation of impatient people in the history of our planet, America here and now is it. This is where the clash comes in, because Tantra, like rising dough or a new pregnancy, can't be rushed. Tantra, when applied to the American mentality, teaches patience, discipline, and inner calm. It shows us not only how, but also where and when to stop and smell the roses. If there was ever a nation that needed that lesson, it's America in the 21st century.

Mental outlook and physical energy are equal in their impact on personal growth. We call the internal side of the meditative, philosophical aspect of Tantra "Right Handed" Tantra. We call the external, physical, energy-raising exercises "Left Handed" Tantra. This book explains the physical part of moving energy through the body, while the exercises keep your attention focused on the training, effectively doing both Right and Left handed Tantra at the same time. It's up to you, the student of the path, to figure out what works best for you.

As for lectures on "safe sex," this seems to be the next popular wave of publicly acceptable sex discussion. I assume that those who read this book have heard all about condoms, sexually transmitted diseases, AIDS, Herpes, etc. You don't need that lecture from me here. Anyone who digs far enough into Tantra will find that fluid exchange is also an important part of Tantra; a part that doesn't work for 21st century Americans. The solution, we've found, is to bless your safe sex tools, --sacred condoms! --which I get into in Chapter 9.

I call this system "American Tantra" not because I invented American Tantra, but because someone has to put it down as a system at some point. If the eastern gurus are going to disdain and criticize us, we'll give them something solid and physical to bash. In future editions of this book, I may include their comments as well, to aid the student in discovering exactly what aspects of American Tantra work, and what will be forgotten in history like the Edsel.

Tantra in America

In researching this book, I dug into some of the mythology of America. Our common mythology gives Americans a basis for a common philosophy that binds us together as a nation. Ideals like freedom, justice, equality, capitalism and political asylum weave together in a tapestry that nobody believes in 100%, but we all pretend to uphold at least a part of it to keep society moving forward.

Like every other population in history, as long as we are whitewashed by our own mythology, we will continue to believe we are free, equal, and prospering, even as our rights and environment erode in front of us. As long as those in power show us that Freedom and Liberty are still in their places of power and still working their particular mojo, we will be agreeable with whatever philosophy they say goes with it. Or will we?

There's this odd human instinct that motivates us to be better than someone else. In America, with our freedom, equality, and justice mythology, we find ourselves penned in by competition and power-over games. No matter how 'equal' we try to be, there are always people in positions of power and authority, and people who are not.

Tantra in America sits in direct opposition to those in power who understand our American mythology and are not afraid to use it against us. As American Tantrics, we are practicing here, (America) and now, (21st century) to become even greater than what those in power want us to become, and to show the rest how it's done. Tantra gives us a way to use our physical bodies to regain the power of Freedom that is our legacy.

> Blue Tantra:
> A new variety of Tantra that includes more than 2 people.

Tantra is also about connecting with another person in a way unlike any other. American Tantra, with its "Blue Tantra" approach, lends itself to groups, families, and communities connecting with each other as well as couples. Once you get to know your housemates, coven-mates, adopted family, or close knit group of friends on a more personal basis, you understand each other on a level that makes peace, love, and joy inevitable. American Tantra is about real Equality, and real Freedom. Freedom of body, mind, spirit, and community.

Who is this writer anyway?

Like all true Americans, I'm a mixed up kid. My mother's side of the family came from Irish immigrants from the 1800's, with some

German and a heavy dose of Native American stock. My father immigrated to this country in the 1940's, due to political unrest in his native Hungary. They met, married, and generated 4 offspring before 1970. When my parents divorced a few years into the 70's, my mother moved the kids out to the country to live with a commune of magicians and Wiccans, which is where my spiritual philosophy was installed.

I was first drawn to Tantra at the age of 14. I understood what sex was supposed to be, on a philosophical and emotional level. I understood the sacredness of the act, watching the adult lovers around me on the farm being open about their sexuality. However, my limited experience with boys my age had turned out quite contrary to what I saw on the commune. When I approached my favorite elder "auntie" about the subject, she laughed and told me to learn Tantra before I hurt myself. When I pressed her about the subject, she said not to sleep with anyone I didn't love, and that made sense, so I dropped the subject. But the word "Tantra" stayed in the back of my head, for the next 10 years.

When I grew up and began exploring different spiritual paths, there was a push to do something different than what my parents had done. My father was still a Lutheran, and Christianity just didn't seem right to me. Since my mother identified with Ceremonial Magick, I began studying Buddhism and eastern philosophy, finding it more fitting to my personality. I wanted to find the oldest written religion on the planet. And there was that word again. Tantra. Synonymous with Sex-magick in some texts, denounced as dangerous or elevated to the highest regard in others.

I set about learning everything I could about the subject. There are many books written on the subject, however, I have been told that most of the ancient ones are in what is called "twilight language", or a metaphor-filled language that sounds very poetic and romantic, but which hide the actual physical facts of the rites. For this reason, it is said that eventually, all students on a true Tantric path must have a physical teacher. However, there is much one can learn before one actually finds a physical teacher, as I learned before I found my teacher. Although we didn't work together very long on the physical, he is still around for me to ask questions of on the internet.

I began teaching Tantra when I opened a small bookstore in the Pacific Northwest. Many solo practitioners wanted to learn, gather knowledge, and make connections with others who were practicing Tantra. This book is an outflow of that information.

Today I have a Masters degree in mental health counseling, an office practice, and a reputation for good classes and workshops. I'm an ordained and licensed High Priestess in the temple of Mystic Arts Gathering and Information Circle (M.A.G.I.C.), and a festival co-coordinator for the Spiral Rhythms Festival. I've got a handfasted mate, two teenage kids, and a community of loving friends that keeps growing.

How to use this book

I have based this book on classroom work, and each lesson has its appropriate homework, or groundwork. The groundwork is broken into three types of exercises: Red, White, and Blue. Red and White are traditional names for certain styles of practice; there is honestly no such thing as Blue Tantra. However, I designed the Blue exercises to accomplish them in groups of three or more.

The meditations are set aside so that you can make photocopies of them to take into temple or on the go with you. These meditations become second nature after a few practices, but at first, the question "am I doing this right" is best answered immediately by looking at a printed copy in front of you. I give you some student stories and examples of how Tantra can affect daily life in little text boxes, too.

I highly recommend that every student dig into the bibliography

> Meditation:
> The act of focusing on one idea, excluding all else.

of this work, and the bibliographies of the works found in my bibliography. With internet technology, most of this is now widely available, which is in sharp contrast to when I began my studies in the '80's. When in doubt, 'Google' it.

Same sex couples are totally capable of utilizing these methods. If you understand that "lingam" is anything that has the same use as "penis" (hands, dildos, toys) and

> Yoni: Sanskrit word for Female genitalia. Also can be applied to any body opening.

"yoni" includes all orifices (vagina, anus, mouth) these meditations make sense.

If you keep up with the groundwork, the ending chapters will

> **Lingam:**
> the Sanskrit word for Penis. Also is applied to any upright object that could be symbolically a penis.

make much more sense. It's possible to get through this book and all of it's assignments in 6 months (without cheating or skipping ahead!) but the average time is approximately 3 years.

Three years? Yes, three whole years. You don't become a master chef by watching one cooking show on TV, and you won't master Tantra by reading one book. So, now is a good time to ask yourself: do you really want to change your life? Or do you just want to "dabble" in something that might be interesting?

This book will satisfy dabblers until about chapter 4. After that, if you don't do the groundwork, the path won't make much sense. If I have just described your situation, just read as far as you need to, then put the book on your shelf till it calls to you again. If you are supposed to study American Tantra, this path will still be here when you're ready.

If, however, you're ready to change your life, you're in for an amazing 3 years.

Chapter 1:   Pranayama and Karezza:

Pranayama

In Sanskrit, Prana means "energy," Yama means "breath." Therefore, Pranayama is energy breath. Breathing, which humans do over 126,000 times a day, is the first thing we do when we leave the womb. This is the beginning of our love/hate relationship with our existence.

The author Osho says that Prana is conatined in the air, just like wetness is contained in water. We can't stop breathing because our sense of survival will force us to inhale eventually. How do you know someone is dead? They stop breathing. However, when the air is not good, we can't breathe correctly and a host of problems occur.

Breathing correctly adds oxygen to the bloodstream, changes the tone of your muscles, and allows all of your cells to function at their best capacity. When there is not enough oxygen in your body, it shuts down unnecessary systems to keep necessary systems alive. This is why, when we don't breathe correctly, such as the moment right before orgasm, our brains only think in loops. There's no energy to expand our thinking. We show ourselves the same mental scenes over and over until we take a big breath, then the thought pattern changes. This often keeps people from being able to orgasm at all.

The same thing is true when we are angry or crying. We think in loops, replaying the scene that caused us pain, because we are not breathing correctly. Once we start breathing correctly again, we can break the loops. Try it sometime. If you always breathe correctly, you'll find yourself in these mindsets much less often.

The ancient Gurus listened to the sound that their Pranayama would make, and they defined that sound as a mantra, (usually a repeated word, or chant) that our minds hear every day, thousands of times a day. They hear the in breath as "Ham" and the exhale as "Sah". Together, Ham-Sah is the

> Pranayama: Breathing exercise that translates literally into "Energy Breath."

mantra of Pranayama. The in breath and exhale....Ham and Sah, Ham–Sah, is a very simple mantra. Stop and listen to it for yourself. Can you hear Ham-Sah?

Many people don't really breathe, but merely sip air, just enough to keep them functioning, but not really alive. These people tend to be very uptight and stressed out. Tell an upset person to breathe, and something will change in them. How well do you breathe? Let's find out; it's time to pay attention to your breath.

Exercise: Pranayama

First, breathe normally. You may notice that the air comes in through your nose, goes down your throat, and into your lungs, and then comes right back out again. Breathe a little deeper. See if you can double the time you spend on each inhale and exhale. Take a moment to try it.

Got that? Good. Now fill your lungs entirely on each inhale and each exhale. Count as you inhale and then again as you exhale. Is one shorter than the other? Slow down the shorter one and stretch it out so that inhale time and exhale time are the same. Remember to use your entire lungs. Take a moment to adjust to this deeper breathing before you move on with this exercise.

Ok, next step is to use your diaphragm to help you open up your lungs further. Most people squeeze their diaphragm upwards as they suck in their stomachs on an inhale. As your stomach comes in, it leaves less room in your chest for air. Reverse that by extending your stomach outward as you inhale, and allowing it to go back to normal on the exhale. It might feel "backward," but keep breathing deeply! You may notice yourself getting light headed after a few breaths...this is normal. You are pumping more oxygen into your brain than you were before, so your brain has to get used to it first. Don't worry; it goes away after a minute or two.

Now that you are breathing deeply and using your diaphragm to the best of your ability, you are pumping more oxygen into your body, and you may even feel your muscles relaxing a bit. To capitalize on that relaxation and to make the most of the oxygen that is now coming into your system, you need to keep that air in your lungs long enough to complete the exchange of gases inside of you. Slow your breathing waaaaaaaaaay down.....very very very slow. So s l o w that it's hardly noticeable. Count the inhale and exhale again, making sure they are the same length. You might find yourself counting all the way to 20. This is excellent.

Focus:

Now for the visualization part. The air you are inhaling is different from the air you are exhaling; the chemical components change inside our lungs. Use your mind's eye to "see" the Prana entering your body as one color, and the Prana leaving your body as another color. Bring one color—perhaps silver or white—in through your nose, straight up and around the inside of your skull, and then down your neck and back to the bottom of your spine. As you exhale, watch as the second color—perhaps gold or gray—takes the same path in reverse; up the spine, across the inside of the crown, past the third eye, and out the nose. This has the effect of making you very aware of your spine.

This slow, deep, diaphragm based breathing will help keep you calm in times of stress, relax you after a hard day, and free your mind of the negative loops it can get into. The color visualization will keep you focused on internal effects, leaving the outside world alone. During your ordinary day, when you catch yourself stressed and not breathing, take a moment to slow down and do pranayama. All other exercises stem from the ability to do pranayama automatically. Once you are comfortable with the depth and slowness of Pranayama, and the focus of the colors changing, you can start correcting for smoothness, long pauses, depth, and noise. A true Pranayama is clean, clear, and smooth. Practice this until it becomes second nature to you.

How is breathing this way going to enhance your sex life? In several different ways. Oxygen content of your blood stream goes up. Sometimes as much as 50%. This changes the way you metabolize EVERYTHING,

> Vibration:
> The result of the energy in your system.
> Healthier people vibrate at a higher rate than unhealthy people do.

which makes you healthier as a whole. Also, when you breathe this way, your focus is on your body, which then becomes a habit, which then becomes an increased ability to focus on your body while in the throes of sexual ecstasy. This type of breathing also straightens your posture and forces the Prana to move correctly through your system. This adds energy to all of your bodily organs, but especially any organs getting your intense attention, like genitals.

Exercise: Attention on Breath

Pay attention to how you are breathing now, and at random times through your day. Make sure your breath is smooth, with no long pauses in between inhale and exhale, and that you are making little or no noise in breathing. Breathe as deeply as you possibly can, feel your breath in your nostrils. Now figure out which side you are breathing more predominantly on, left or right. Make note of it in your journal for a week. What do you notice? What does that mean?

The 28 minute threshold

Neurologists have found that the human brain uses both hemispheres for different reasons, and switches back and forth regularly. At any given moment, we are using the majority of functions on

> 28 minutes:
> The time it takes for your brain to switch modes from Right brained thinking to left brained thinking or vice-versa.

one side or the other. Our left brain houses our language centers, our right brain deals more with with spatial orientation. The average amount of time a human spends focused in either hemisphere is about 28 minutes, with an in-between transfer time of about 4 to 5 minutes. This is an organic process, so of course it isn't sudden. It is during these times that we have our most inspiring thoughts and solutions to problems.

If you do pranayama breathing and continue for about 28 minutes, you will be accessing both sides of your brain, and at the same time, making the most of your mental energy. This is what we refer to as having a balanced mindset. When you have reached this balanced mindset once, it becomes easier and easier to achieve in later tries. You are prana-charging your brain at these moments, and this exercise changes everything in your system.

A Cancer Survivor's Story:
"J" was a 68-year-old man when he took my class. He was just diagnosed with early prostate cancer. As he went through the typical radiation treatment to destroy a small tumor, he would begin pranayama as soon as he was comfortable on the treatment table.. A strange warmth would envelop his whole pelvic region, even before the treatment started. As the staff moved around him to do their jobs, "J" would step out of his ordinary mindset in a daydream/astral sort of way. It was in this mindset that he came to the conclusion to radically change his diet. Eating only raw foods and fresh juices, as well as his Pranayama meditations on the radiation table, he kicked the cancer in less than a year, and remains cancer-free eight years later. He still juices and does pranayama every day and has a host of astounded doctors.

The Clock Trick:

Whenever you have a timed meditation, turn your back on the clock. Literally. If you are able to simply open your eyes and see what time it is, you will be tempted to do so every two or three minutes. If you have the clock at your back so that you must make a concerted effort to pull yourself back to the physical world and turn your entire body around, you will be more inclined to push yourself farther before you turn to see how long you have been meditating. If you can't put your back to the clock, turn the clock's face away from you.

The idea is to push yourself beyond your previous meditation time. Not knowing the time should make you push yourself farther. Coax yourself beyond what you "think" you did, and you will be surprised at your perceptions of time.

Groundwork:

-White: Practice Pranayama for at least 28 minutes, and discover the balanced mindset powered by extra Prana and the Right/Left shift. Get comfortable with this exercise so that it becomes second nature. To master this exercise, you should be able to drop into the balanced mindset within 10 breaths.

-Red: Practice Pranayama for at least 28 minutes as a couple while laying facing each other, with your clothes on. Try to time the in breaths and out breaths together. If this leads to removal of clothing and or eventual sex, wait until you have accomplished 28 minutes of breathing together first. You may find that even during sex, you will feel drawn to breathing together.

-Blue: Practice Pranayama with a group of people sitting in a circle facing each other. Watch how the other people in the circle breathe, and have everyone try to match each other as well as stretch out the breath longer each time. If you can continue this for 28 minutes, allow the group to relax and drift as long as they need to afterward.

How exciting!

The peripheral (or below-the-neck) nervous system has two types of signals it can send: Excitatory signals and inhibitory signals. When you bend your elbow, some signals are saying "Expand" and some signals are saying "contract" because that's what has to happen with the two sets of front and back arm muscles.

Tantra begins with the nerve endings in your body. Each muscle group has the ability to move due to messages coming from your brain saying either "excite" (flex) or "inhibit" (relax). The extra energy from Tantra comes from simultaneously activating the "excite" and "inhibit" commands of each nerve cell. It is important to know how to both "excite" and "inhibit" your own musculature and, as a result, your own neurons. This is what will give you that extra energy boost in Tantra.

What happens when you simultaneously "excite" and "inhibit" the same neuron? What happens when you add Pranayama to that equation, or better yet, add the excite/inhibit formula to Pranayama?

The result is an exercise known to most as "Karezza," developed by Alice Bunker Stockham in the late 1800's. Karezza, which means "caress," is a physical body training exercise that makes an impact in the psyche that affects our sexual centers, as well as every other part of the human anatomy. Learning this exercise will change your entire attitude about sex, and about your own body. This is a big part of what makes Tantra so popular.

When you're sexually aroused, three systems activate simultaneously. These are the nervous system (sensitivity to touch), the circulatory system (heart rate, blood flow to certain tissues), and muscle tension (arching your back and tensing your thighs). Karezza is about learning to control these three major systems during sexual arousal. Why do we want to control these systems? Better sex, of course!

When you have sex--even masturbation--there are three things at work. The muscle system makes your body tense up. The circulatory system speeds up to use up oxygen, and the mind goes into loops that release hormones that make our nerve endings more sensitive. When orgasm happens during ordinary sex, all three of those systems "snap." They get all the energy they are going to get. The muscles can't get any tenser, the oxygen can't be used up any faster, the hormones are all released, the skin is as sensitive as it can get. Letting go of that maximum potential gives us that familiar feeling of orgasm, and the resulting release of fluids is the intended result.

Immediately afterward, these three systems go into their recovery mode. However, when you control all of these systems by relaxing the muscles, breathing deeply and slowly, and

> Masturbation:
> Do-it-yourself sex.

staying away from the hormone releasing thought patterns, you are simultaneously triggering the excitatory and inhibitory potentials of all of your nerves. You are telling your muscles to contract and relax at the same time. You are controlling the amount of oxygen in the circulatory system, and the amount of hormones released. Orgasmic feelings tend to last longer, take less time to recover afterward, and in many instances, the resulting orgasm is more intense. When done correctly, it can even prevent orgasm from happening at all. This is why Alice Stockham first introduced it to America; to use as birth control!

Under the act of Karezza, the energy of the orgasm seems to "backfire" through the nervous system, spreading out to nerves that typically would never encounter a charge of that magnitude. The relaxation of the muscles, nerves, and chemistry allows the energy to spread out across the entire system. We harness this energy when we practice Tantra with—and without—a partner.

Being here now

Up until this exercise, you have been having sex on autopilot. One of these three systems--nervous system, blood-flow system, or muscle system-- gets going, and then the other two jump right up and start their thing too. When practicing Tantra, one must be in total control of all three systems, so that your body doesn't become a runaway train when participating in Tantra.

One concept I'll introduce you to is the "be here now" philosophy of sex. Most people check out with what I call "pocket fantasies." These are those fantasies that are right there in the pocket when you need one. Most people need a fantasy to get off sexually. If you pay attention to what is going on with your body here and now, you should not need to use fantasy for sexual turn-ons. If you are getting a blowjob and fantasizing about how good it would be if only she would do a certain particular thing, you're not paying attention to how great it is now. Get rid of the fantasies by focusing on how good sex feels here and now. That takes a unique sort of discipline.

> Pocket fantasy:
> A fantasy that you use regularly to get yourself into a more intense state of sexual arousal. The "pocket fantasy" works every time you need to use it.

Compare your orgasm to climbing up a mountain: You get increasingly high on the vibration, and then, suddenly, you get to the highest peak and go over the edge of the cliff into orgasm.

Fantasy takes your energy away from that goal. You go halfway up the mountain, then suddenly take a shortcut over the edge. It leads your attention to things that are not on this plane of existence, and deposits your energies there. Does your favorite celebrity really need your extra energy?

The idea behind Karezza (and Tantra) is to get to that highest erotic peak and

> Karezza:
> A meditation that involves self-stimulation and bodily control. This becomes a clearing tool for negative energy.

hang out there, without going over the edge of the cliff into the orgasm, for as long as humanly possible.

Why? Because that is the point of sex. What's the point of sex? To connect-- to become One with another. Do you want that ecstasy of being One with your partner for only 10 seconds, or would you rather connect for hours on end? To have the orgasm makes it end rather abruptly and immediately. Pack up your toys and go home.

The point of Karezza practice, which includes pranayama to control the circulatory system and the "be here now" philosophy to control your hormone releases, is to train your body to keep that orgasmic energy built up. This leads to a rise in your vibration and a connection with One that is meditative. To hang on the edge of the cliff for as long as possible is what you need to reach that vibrational state we call "enlightenment."

If, however, you do this exercise and find yourself vibrating too high, or you're too energized, or you're antsy or anxious, try the following:

> Enlightenment:
> The state of mind that is the goal of most spiritual pursuits. The concept of knowing all that must be known to transcend one's own karma.

Exercise: Grounding

Visualize roots growing from your feet into the ground. If you can't 'see' them, then feel them. Allow them to sink as far into the ground as you can. Then, take a deep breath, and as you exhale, let the energy in your system sink through your body, down the roots, and into the earth. Repeat as necessary, or until you feel better.

Controlling the orgasm

There is an Eastern tradition that gives men intense training in how to withhold their ejaculation during an orgasmic climax. They equate male semen to Prana, and its loss

> Ejaculation:
> The fluids ejected from the body--both male and female--during sex.

signifies a loss of energy for the male. There were complicated tricks developed to allow men to learn how to control their orgasm and not ejaculate, or, even more difficult, to recover the semen after it has been ejaculated by use of a graduated training method. Men who practiced this exercise learned to absorb the ejaculate back into the penis using only their muscles. They would start with water, then graduate to milk, then on to olive oil, then even thicker liquids like honey. This would take years of painful and annoying practice, all due to a belief in the connection of semen to Prana.

We know from experience in the West that a man's body continues to create sperm all through his life, whether he expels it or not, and that his vigor has nothing to do with the amount of sperm expelled. However, this sort of ejaculate control still has a place in Tantra, as I'll explain in a moment.

Orgasm DOES equate with an energetic release, if not a loss, so I recommend that all students, male and female, learn to control their orgasms by learning to withhold them, or put them off as long as possible. You can conserve the energy expended in the muscle contractions and vocalizations during orgasm and use it in Tantra, if you don't toss it out during sex. The decision of whether or not to expend that orgasmic energy is up to you, however, you should be informed of it's effects both negative and positive.

Female orgasm is no different from male orgasm in this respect; energy expended during orgasm can come in handy later on, so conservation is a good idea anytime, even if it isn't entirely withholding orgasm. What confuses and concerns many women when they begin Tantra are the copious amounts of vaginal fluids that arise from Tantric sex, including the Karezza exercise. This is quite normal, and is actually advantageous for long sexual encounters such as advanced Tantric penetration, so there is no need to be concerned. Simply make sure your water consumption is optimal.

Exercise: Karezza

One of my students coined the term "Masterbatitation" for this exercise, and a very fitting one it is. Technically, this is "Karezza." This is also the groundwork for this lesson:

Do this exercise when you are alone. Put yourself in a sacred space where you will not be bothered for at least an hour. Your private bedroom is the perfect place for this meditation. Light candles and incense as a reminder that this is a sacred act.

Lay down on your bed nude. Relax every muscle in your body;

go limp like a rag doll. Get into the Pranayama breathing pattern, and allow your mind to drift into the space you found earlier when you practiced. Focus on the here and now. Using very little physical effort, begin masturbating. Use lubrication if you must, but not large amounts. Slowly, using one hand only, stimulate yourself, paying close attention to all of your body systems. Relax and just experience the feeling of your hand on your genitals. Don't drop into your typical fantasizing mind trip, and don't try to imagine that there is another person in the room. Just experience your own hand giving yourself pleasure, and tell yourself "this is the experience of masturbation." Keep your breathing slow and regulated. Keep all of your muscles relaxed; let your body become limp,, moving only what you need to stay sexually aroused. Focus on the pleasure in your genitals.

When you feel yourself becoming aroused, keep in mind that you should be relaxed. The energy caused in your genitals will spread across your entire body if you stay relaxed. Keep the Pranayama going too. Whenever you feel yourself getting distracted, focus on a small area of your genitals and bring yourself back. Relax and focus is the game.

Your body will want to tense up; make it relax by letting go of the energy from your groin. Breathe. Spread it out to the rest of your body to energize it. Allow yourself to hang on the edge of that cliff for as long as you can. You may notice that it's sort of like waves on the beach, rushing and crashing and rushing again.... back off when you think you need to, relax, re-center yourself, and continue. You want to stay in this state for as long as you can.

Relax and breathe as your desire builds. If you find yourself on the verge of the cliff that is orgasm, stop masturbating and breathe deeply. Try to stay aroused but not orgasmic—staying on the edge of the cliff—for at least 28 minutes.

One strategy that works is to build up and back off repeatedly for 28 minutes. If you accidentally go over the cliff into orgasm, look at the time on the clock (when you're grounded again!) and consider it your "best time" and try to...uhm... beat it next time. Do not chide yourself for failure in these exercises ever! It will not work to train yourself to avoid orgasm by focusing on baseball scores, ugly people, or anything else that might turn you off; you must truly gain control of your own biological systems. If you orgasm beyond the 28 minute mark, allow that energy to propel you into your imagination for as long as you can lie there. Post-orgasm is the time where fantasy can have its lead. This is also great practice for astral travel.

If you make it to that 28-minute window, your body will change and orgasm will no longer be an issue. You will find yourself floating in a strange, indescribable fashion. However, this float is useful for receiving psychic information and other important things. Don't be in a hurry to return.

This meditation takes practice and patience. I don't know many who have achieved 28 minutes in less than three attempts. Personally, it took me five. So, be patient.... it's worth it.

Once you get into the habit of being in this headspace when you are masturbating, you will be able to do the same thing with a lover. Many times we are afraid that if our lover doesn't sense us tense up and thrust when he/she strokes us just so, our lover may not be getting the correct message that what they are doing is pleasant. You can correct for this by making your wishes known verbally. Hearing "yeah, do that!" is more accurate than tensing up and thrusting anyway. When you use this method in a couples setting, it makes it much easier to verbalize what you want.

Working Karezza in a solo fashion teaches you to give your body exactly what it asks for. You can touch yourself in a way that can only be discerned from within, which gives you the opportunity to love yourself.

A Virgin's Dilemma;

"P," a beautiful but shy 20-year-old girl, sat quietly through the lecture on this topic, not asking a whole lot of questions till the end of class.

After class, she pulled me aside and explained that she had never had an orgasm, and in fact, had never had sex. From all the attempts she had made at masturbation, she had never reached climax, and feared that she was 'frigid.' I suggested she go ahead and try the groundwork. A week later, after attempting this exercise

---

for over 60 minutes with no results, she feared that she would need to drop the class.

I advised her to try again, utilizing the most "out there" masturbation methods that she could think of. I gave her specific permission to use the pocket fantasy until she had overcome this hurdle. I suggested that she go all out and pursue any type of solo sexual activity that she had ever thought of. I also recommended toys, groups, and websites for her.

A month later (and very behind in her lessons) she emailed me telling me that she managed to achieve an orgasm. She had installed a shower massage unit, and used that to relax all the muscles in her genitals. Then, stepping out of the shower and immediately utilizing two vibrators in accordance with a stifled fantasy she had always had, she was able to bring herself to climax. Not only that, but she was able to accomplish this chapter's groundwork less than a week later. All she needed was 'permission' within herself to follow that fantasy, and releasing that energy allowed her to continue with the lessons."

She discovered that her supposed "frigidity" was based in her shyness and fear of social contacts. Karezza helped shake this to the surface for her. "P" now has a flourishing sex life with a steady partner, and has overcome the worst of her shyness.

Experience is everything

Experience is a large part of Tantra. Not experience, but Experience, with a capital E. The difference is in the methods used to Experience or experience. When you are driving through a very beautiful area, you are experiencing the view. When you stop the car, get out, sit down on the grass and breathe it all in, you are Experiencing the entire place. Everything in life is an Experience. We're born on this planet with a physical body so that we can use it to have a real human Experience. Experience includes eating, smelling, touching, seeing, and hearing. Most of what we consider to be human experience is actually just the thoughts in our heads, the emotions we encounter, and our reactions to it, not actual physical reality. When we Experience reality, we pay more attention to the fun we are having. This makes all the difference when you apply it to the principles of making love.

> Experience:
> When capitalized, Experience is a mindset of paying attention to the here and now with all 5 of your senses.

Many humans experience sex on a small level. They find someone who is attractive enough to make their erectile tissues erect, and proceed into a scripted behavior, designed to convince the other person to have sex. Then, they take this person and use him/her as a life-sized sex toy. By not connecting with the human being inside the body, they treat this living person as if he/she didn't have a spirit. The next day, they don't discuss it any further than compliments in the morning, if the script was done right.

To Experience sex is a totally different ball game. Not only must the person you are attracted to be able to affect your erectile tissue, he/she must also be able to connect with you on some other plane such as shared interests or conversation, and usually more than 3 or 4 separate areas of union need to be present for good sexual Experiences. This other connection makes the Experience happen. This is one reason that many Tantrics are monogamous or limit their partners; it's difficult to find a union like that.

A couple who is into Experiencing sex will not wish to simply view it through the windshield at 55 mph. They have to slow down and take their time, savoring each moment of the act from flirting thru foreplay all the way to cleanup. Usually it starts with a deep look into each other's eyes. There is a recognition from both partners that there is a force bringing them together. To create a good sexual Experience from this base, it's important to be Here and Now, not thinking about future performance or past issues.

Take the energy, focus your attention to each touch, and kiss that your partner bestows upon you. Put all of your attention on the tips of your fingers as you run them over your partner's body. Get all of your body involved, not just genitalia.

Finally, the best way to Experience sex is to s-l-o-w d-o-w-n. Remember, the moment you orgasm, a lot of the fun is done. Put that moment off as long as you can by relaxing your muscles and breathing.

Magick and Wicca vs. Tantra

Anyone who is familiar with the work of Aleister Crowley understands that he used much sex magick in his works. In fact, this WWII era British Occultist and author came to rely very heavily on the energy created by the human body during orgasm. Upon examination of the evidence, we find that Crowley had access to higher teachings of the East, most likely Tantra.

Tantra utilizes energy created by the human body, not only during orgasm, but at other times as well. The exercises in Tantra lead one to a total control of the nervous system and hence total control over a person's physical energy. To control the nervous system is to reign in the pleasure response, so that this energy builds up and becomes a useful tool for raising consciousness.

Crowley practiced this variety of Tantra. The correlation that Crowley made was that any energy intense enough to open up consciousness was also intense enough to power magickal spell-work. However, you can't have one without the other. This is something that the Hindus and Taoist and Buddhists understand as Karma.

The similarities between Tantra and CM are numerous: It's best to do them both nude. Both happen sacred space, usually with an altar set up burning incense and candles. Both require a certain amount of understanding of metaphysics before attempting. In addition, both use sexual intercourse in their workings.

The difference between Tantra and C.M. are subtle, but there. Usually Tantra only focuses on two people; CM and Wicca work well with groups. Tantra works with both partners in trance state from the beginning of the rite; CM and Wicca include getting into trance state as part of the rite. Tantra requires all participants be familiar with advanced concepts before the rite begins. CM and Wicca are available for anyone willing to learn the steps of the ritual. Both Wicca and Tantra focus on clearing personal energy, which then leads to physical manifestation. CM leans toward physical manifestation, which then invokes the repercussive spell work (or Karmic lesson) that clears the personal energy.

Tantra teaches not only control of the orgasm, but also how to 'amp it up', how to make it more powerful. In Crowley's day, it was trial and error, experimenting and documenting his own experience. Now, there are much easier ways of learning this control, mostly due to the availability of texts and websites on the subject. This generation of Sex Magickians has everything from Pranayama breathing exercises to complex rites invoking 16 different forms of Shakti, all available over the Internet.

Just because the information is out there doesn't make one a Tantric just by reading it. Nor does reading the entire Golden Dawn library make you a ceremonial magickian. Like any good path, the practice is at the heart of it. If you can understand your Karma, and you understand that there is something for you to learn, Tantra is a useful tool in clearing the psychological barriers to healthy, happy lives.

"An Artist's Ache"

K was a photographer, writer, and dancer who was gaining a reputation of being promiscuous, drinking too much in public, and embarrassing herself and her partner. She came to see me as one of her methods of healing from a systemic disease that was overwhelming her doctors. As I worked with her, I noticed she would "check out" in the middle of listening. She would ask a question, I would give her an answer, but she would be staring blankly at the wall, or looking off into space.

When I talked to her husband about his perspective on her problems, he told me that she often checked out like that at home, and especially whenever he mentioned sex. Their sex life had deteriorated in a short amount of time, after she had returned from a trip to her hometown.

I suggested she do the Karezza exercise, and pay attention to what came up with her. She later said that the Karezza meditation allowed her to recall a short incident that she had blocked from her memory entirely. An old boyfriend who had been abusive in the

---

past again sexually assaulted her during her trip home. Since that time, any inference to sex would cause her to leave her body and float above herself, looking down on whatever scene she was in. With more therapy from other sources, she began to heal from the assault, overcame her health problems, and began living her life like normal again. Without the release of Karezza, she may have fought this mystery battle for many more years.

Groundwork:

White: 28 min Karezza (Masturbatitation described above). Practice at least 2 times before moving on to the exercises in the next chapter.

Red: Full Experience during Sex:
    No, you cannot simply transfer the Karezza exercise from White to Red without further instructions, however....The next time you find yourself in a position to be sexual slow down the action. Be fully in the here and now, and watch what your bodies are doing from the inside. If something feels good, enjoy it for how it feels rather than think "it would feel much better if..." See if the change in focus changes the outcome of the sexual experience for you

Blue: Be Here Now Party
    Throw a party with one rule: the participants may only discuss what is currently going on in front of them. Play games, watch movies, or cook food together, but stipulate that no one may discuss past or future, and no one may discuss anything that is not currently in the room. This isn't as easy as it sounds!

Chapter 2:   Chakras

Right Handed vs. Left Handed Tantra

Traditional schools of thought differentiate between Right Handed (internally focussed) and Left Handed (externally focussed) Tantric techniques. The difference between right handed and left handed Tantra can be described as such: If the ancient texts say "Students who sit in the mud shall receive enlightenment" the Right hand practitioner will contemplate what is meant by "sit" and what is meant by "mud" and why the two are linked together. The Left hand practitioner will go find a puddle and plop his butt into it to find the enlightenment therein. American Tantra can actively use both aspects. We can choose to contemplate the meaning of the words, and/or discover their link by getting our physical selves into the act, not just contemplation of word meanings in twilight language.

When practicing with the earlier exercises, a good thought to tack on the end of the energy release is "show me the information I need before I need it." This sets you up to pay closer attention to the signals and signs that the Universe drops in your lap. It also encourages serendipity magick, which is my way of describing semi-miraculous things that happen because you are in the right place at the right time. This is the combination of Right and Left handed approaches.

The traditional Gurus shudder at the audacity, I'm sure.

The Universal Vibration:

Everything in the Universe is vibrating. The air molecules around you are full of energy. The room around you is full of light waves and sound waves. The combination of all of this ambient energy is Prana.

To make full use of the Prana around you, you must be fully aware of all of it. To be fully aware, you must be fully in the moment. Here. Now. Stop reading this for a moment and check out what is going on around you. Light. Sound. Temperature. Texture of clothing on skin. Feel of air in nostrils, the smells around you....go ahead, stop reading and do this.

Now, check your internal energy levels. What happened when you took that moment to check in with the here and now? You probably feel slightly more awake, slightly more energized. How do you make use of that energy? Be here and now all the time. There is only one point that you can interact with reality, and that is here and now. Past is done, future ain't here yet. If you're driving and thinking about dinner, you're not in the moment. The idea is to expand your awareness so that you are getting the most of the here and now.

If we weren't here to watch sunsets, why do we have eyes engineered to see the colors? The idea is to use the senses of the body, here and now, to increase the joy in our lives, which therefore increases our vibration.

When something is vibrating at its peak level, it is not only at its healthiest state, but also it is in its most joyful state. That goes for humans, racehorses, and amoebas. A healthy human is a happy human. Raising your vibration will increase your level of joy.

The idea of being "here and now" is impossible for some people to grasp due to body-induced memory of traumatic history, so they "check out" of reality. Not so easy for a Tantric, who must stay on top of the energy system and not allow it to be sidetracked like that. If you find yourself "checking out" of reality when really cool stuff is happening (sex, concerts, educational opportunities) do look closer at the reasons why.

Remember the "pocket fantasy?" This is the fantasy that gets you turned on, guaranteed every time. It could be something you've never done, or something you always make a point of doing. It changes for most people from time to time, but basically, it's the fantasy world that is right behind your eyes that you can go to if you need to mentally "check out" while still being able to perform. Tantrics have to retrain themselves OUT of using the pocket fantasy; otherwise, they are not 100% present in the act.

What is going on in front of you better be just as good as anything in your imagination is, or you are wasting your time. The old saying "a bird in the hand is worth two in the bush" might be too cliché here, but it's true. If your reality isn't what you expected it to be, either your expectations are too high, or you're doing something wrong.

Raised vibrational states

Most people can relate to the experience of higher vibrational states, because they have experienced their entire system vibrating like crazy as they got closer to sexual orgasm, giving them that delicious explosion at the end. Sex isn't the only time we feel these raised vibrational tingles, though. When we eat something specifically yummy, when we feel apprehensive about entering a new space, when we realize we have just won something, we get a spontaneous reaction in our bodies that results in a raising of our vibration. This is the joyful, fun part of being human.

However, pain is also a part of being human. Pain can raise our vibration if we know how to handle it. If we don't handle it positively, pain lowers our vibration by creating resistance in our bodies.

You may not believe me now, but here's the secret: the only real pain is the pain of resisting here and now. All other pain is a reminder to do something different. Therefore, if you are in pain, you are resisting something that's happening around you. If release your resistance to what is going on, the source of the pain will heal. Why? Because resistance lowers vibration. Are you resisting or accepting what is going on around you? If you are resisting it, you have labled something "Bad." Look closely at that lable and stop trying to fight off the "bad" part.

The pain here is not just emotional pain, but physical pain, intellectual pain (a.k.a. frustration), grief, and all sorts of other negative situations. Your vibration is also lowered when you are carrying baggage from the past, fears of the future, unmet needs, and a host of other issues. A lot of early White Tantra (solo) work focuses on fixing these issues so that the vibration can go up.

This is another point where Tantra coincides with Ceremonial Magick and Wicca. The Wiccan creed is "An ye harm none, do as ye Will." Ceremonial Magicians word it "Do as Thou Will shall be the Whole of the Law. Love is the Law, Love under Will." They mean the same thing. Being on the right path means doing your Will, walking your correct trajectory through life, having the healthiest vibration you can have.

Getting Naked:

To master Tantra requires taking off all your outer layers to access to the part of our psyche that Sigmund Freud dubbed the "Id". I remember sitting in my psychology lectures in college, thinking, "too bad Sigmund Freud never knew about Tantra." His work with the subconscious would have had much more substance had he had access to the documents of the ancient yogis. As it was, his limited scope allowed the Western world a scientific view of the mechanisms that underlie the science of Tantra.

Freud's "Id" can be translated to the "Atman," "Ka" or "Naked Flame" in Tantra. When you remove all ego and superego masks, you are essentially allowing anything covering the Naked Flame to fall away. The Naked Flame is your True Will plus the energy it takes to manifest your True Will.

Most of the baggage that covers our Naked Flame comes from our upbringing, with a little extra thrown in from our first tight relationships. Many times we don't recognize baggage for what it is, saying to ourselves "that's just the way I am." We call our baggage our 'personality quirks' and think that makes us individually interesting. However, the real YOU inside must be infinitely more interesting than any baggage/quirk you could put on top of it, simply because it is genuine. That fear of heights might be the "way you are," but it's not the real YOU.

The Naked Flame is your divine spark. When you take off all of the masks, fears, and self-imposed boundaries, it is Naked for all the world to see. It's a very powerful state of being. No energy diverts to hold up parts of you that are not real. The Naked Flame also requires that we feed it with experiences. It needs us to open up to the joy of living.

When you remove all masks, your Naked Flame comes into direct contact with the light, air, sound, and other vibrations around you. The world seems brighter, and there is more energy for you to utilize in your own system. To wear nothing on the outside of the Naked Flame is not physically possible with a solid body, but it IS energetically possible. We recognize people who are in that state as more "real" than others and consider them to be "wiser" than most. People who let their masks down are allowing us in, allowing that Naked Flame to do the acting for them, allowing all the energy of this lifetime to go down deep into the source. These people naturally have a happier existence than those who carry the baggage that creates ego masks, and they are usually quite popular in whatever group you find them. If a happier existence isn't enough motivation to let that Naked Flame get free, then what else could there be?

The ancients had many ways of removing masks and baggage. Some ancient techniques that still work are Hatha yoga, transcendental meditation, austerity and intentional poverty, ecstatic dance, rhythm-induced trances, sensory deprivation, mind altering substances, fasting and celibacy. These methods work because they take the student out of every day mindset and puts him or her in a place where they can access the deeper recesses of the subconscious. These techniques force the student to gain control over at least one of the three denizens of existence: body, mind, or actions.

Celibacy, fasting, and other methods of deprivation add energy to the system by not expending it. You simultaneously desire and

> Celibacy:
> The act of not releasing any energy in a sexual fashion, including masturbation

resist the urge to eat, to consume goods, to participate in society, or to have sex. This push-pull mindset allows energy to build up behind a chakra. It will be energy of your own choosing, going when and how you need to put it. When you simultaneously approach and resist an energy force, even if that is your own hunger, then you have a motor in which to crank up energy. You have that magnetism that spins the flywheel inside your own body that can create an energy force to work with.

The trick is to spread it across your entire physical body, allowing the localized energy to mellow into a more generalized form that stretches from your toes to the tips of your hair. When this happens, you will toss off any masks associated with this surrender/resistance pull. You will correct your diet, your social life, or your sexuality issues.

To connect your energy with another person, it is imperative that you give up all masks, and to do that, you must see the masks first. All of these methods work for this purpose, which is why they have persisted all these years. Most are found in some form in all cultures.

When using these traditional methods, recognize that many people have gone before you and have much to say about the subject. Do your homework on whichever method you are choosing, finding a good teacher when necessary. I always recommend that when messing with your own psychology, whether it is through fasting, use of mind-altering substances, or intentional poverty, always have a "spotter", someone who is not participating but who knows what is going on. This way, if you should truly scare yourself, harm yourself, or program yourself with a bigger problem, someone will know the method you took to get there. No tradition anywhere allows an untrained student access to higher states of awareness without a spotter of some kind.

Attention:

Learning to focus can feel like the most tedious, boring, and unnatural thing for an American. However, it becomes much more interesting when you realize this simple truth: Energy flows where attention goes. Wherever you put your attention is where you are putting your energy.

Think about the things you think about. How often are you giving your attention to things you would rather not put energy into? If you begin watching what you are watching, and spending your time and attention like you spend your money, you'll notice a difference.

If you have ever felt drained after having what is jokingly termed a "pity fuck," you understand what I mean. If the person you are having sex with is depressed, hurt, or grieving, you may notice a lowered energy after sex. Your attention was on that person, and your energy flowed that direction. You may even have given them that sexual attention on purpose to help them feel better.

If you find yourself daydreaming about someone you've had sex with, you may have given yourself an accidental link. simply by the amount of attention you are pouring into the link. If you want the link to thrive, continue the daydreaming. If, however, you'd rather have annoying daydreams go away, simply stop putting attention on that person. The energy source for them will wither and die. Training your attention requires persistence and drive.

Take a look at how you are living. Are there things that take more time and energy in your life than they are worth? Do you spend more time trying to pay for things you want rather than enjoying the things you have? Are you giving your attention/energy away to inanimate objects, like calendars and clocks?

If so, simplify. Think critically about the items you spend time working on or working to pay for. If you don't truly need those things, get rid of them. Those are things you won't have to do maintenance on, work for, or worry about having stolen. If you truly get nothing back from a particular friendship, stop trying. Get rid of time wasters, cut back on the number of deadlines you live by, remove the clutter. Give yourself space to breathe.

How To Focus:

Exercise: Fruit and Flowers Experience

Get an apple from any local source. Wash it and place it on your altar. Get a fresh carnation flower—white is best—and rinse it under water, too, then place it on your altar. Get some chocolate--a little bite size piece. Put that on your altar too.

Sit in front of the altar and breathe deeply. Set your breathing with Pranayama.

Now closely examine the apple. Pick it up and look at it from every angle. Take the time to notice every bump, spot, and stripe on its surface. Ask yourself "what makes this apple different from all other apples?" Now rub it on your cheek and feel the texture of its skin. Tell yourself "This is the experience of feeling an apple." Smell it, allow whatever memories come to you from the scent of it. Think of the sunshine and earth minerals that are in this apple. Take your time and savor every sensory organ you have as it applies to this apple. Now take a tiny bite of it. Slowly chew and let the flavor soak in with the message "this is the experience of an apple." Feel it to your very soul. Eat the apple in this fashion, making sure to take note of every bite. Have you ever had an apple quite like this? Sex is not the only thing that can be sensuous.

Now pick up the flower. Adding sensory input you would typically not use, examine the flower the same way you examined the apple. Look at the shape and color of the flower and it's components. Feel how the petals affect your skin sensations. Smell the flower deeply. Tell yourself "This is the experience of a carnation." Now gently pluck one petal from the flower and put it in your mouth. Taste the flower petal, and recognize that this is a sensation you would not normally get, if you were to keep to the "norm" of what you consider is do-able with a carnation. Now smell the flower again; did you get more out of it the second time, after adding the sensation of taste? This is how our bodies work; the more sensory organs we get involved in the processing of an experience, the more we get out of our experiences in general.

Now for the chocolate...focusing on a very small part of your body, the tip of your tongue, imagine that your entire body shrinks to that one small area. All of your nerve endings connect to the ones on the tip of your tongue. When you feel that you are as focused on that area as you possibly can be, put the chocolate on your tongue and let it melt. Allow that feeling and flavor to be everything to you right now. Can you translate that feeling thru your body? Can you feel that chocolate running down your back, down your arms and legs? Practice the focusing exercise until you can.

There are many ways to incorporate sensation into regular activities. Anytime you have conversations, quench thirst or hunger, travel through a landscape, or simply watch the environment, you can incorporate more of our senses into the experience, and get more out of our lives. How many forgotten apples have you eaten? This is the part of Tantra that is Hedonistic, the part that wallows in the sheer joy of being alive.

We only have 24 hours in any given day. We only have 365 days in any given year. We only have—at best—100 years on the planet. We can't extend that time yet, but we can make the most out of it. If you are not using 100% of your sensory organs at least 50% of the time, you're definitely missing something.

Why Chakra Work Helps Raise Vibration:

Kundalini meditations are the cornerstone of Tantric practice. In ordinary waking life, we can sometimes feel traces of the Kundalini energy in our systems, with neat little affects such as shivers up the spine, or muscles that tick. Active Kundalini is one of the greatest energy highs ever! To activate this

> Kundalini:
> A meditation based in breath and visualizations. This becomes a tool for chakra clearing.

amazing energy, there are breathing meditations that take the energy from the sexual center, up the spine, and move it through the rest of the body. When you activate Kundalini, you can create an energy field that combines with that of your partner. To get to this point, you have to go through some intense mental acrobatics--clearing out old emotional baggage, and the energy that messes up the rest of the physical body. This is called Chakra clearing.

W.T.F. is a Chakra?

Chakras are psychic energy organs, designed to give and receive energy from our environment to the various areas in our nervous system. You can visualize them like a whirlpool in your aura, pulling energy inward like a drain pulling water. In Eastern Tantra, there are seven recognized main chakras, with secondary chakras on the hands and feet, and even smaller ones throughout the body. Some estimate over 144,000 chakras on one physical body! You won't have to know them all, just the 7 main ones for now.

When a chakra is blocked or stuck, that means it's filled with energy and not working correctly. The whirlpool is stopped. This can lead to reacting to situations instead

> Chakra:
> A whirlpool in your aura that pulls in energy from your environment. There are 7 major chakras on the human body.

of acting on situations, and you wind up a victim of your surroundings, rather than a willing player in the game of life. It's this chakra clearing that makes Tantra such a powerful force for change.

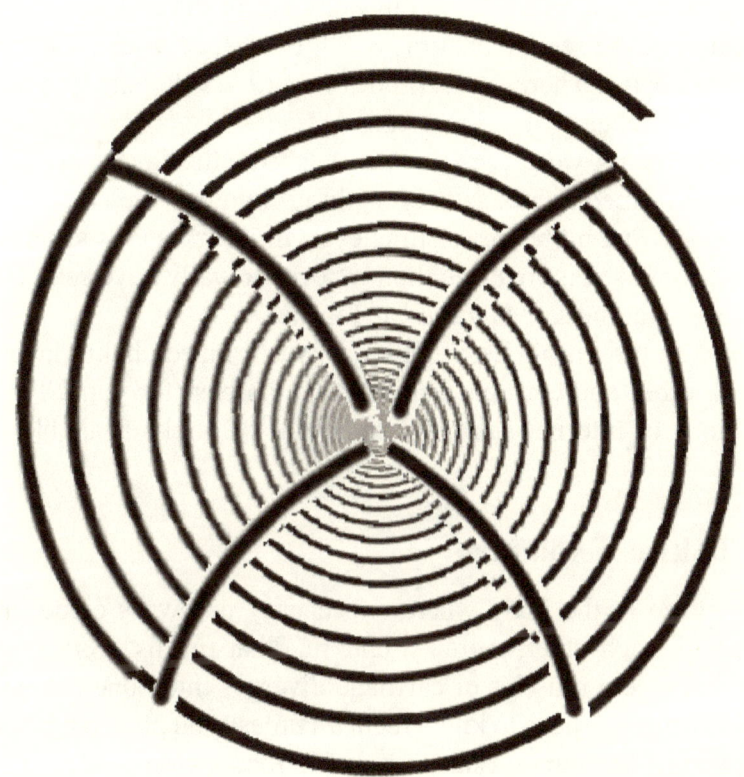

Chakras are like whirlpools, pulling in energy.

So, where is that pesky sex chakra?

There are different systems you will find in books about Chakras. Most of them will give you the Sanskrit names of the chakras. I don't think it's necessary to know their names in a different language to know what they do. Besides, learning the Sanskrit is distracting. Therefore, I have given them American English names, but you might find them called by their numbers (#1 being on the bottom) or colors. It truly doesn't matter what you call them or what colors you assign to them. What matters is where they are located in the body.

There is a tendency in America to swap the two bottom chakras, "sex" and "stability." If you ask Any American on the street, "Where do you feel your sex drive?" they're not going to tell you that they feel it in their abdomen. They'll say that between their legs, where the base chakra resides, is where they feel their sexual urges. However, most of the reproductive materials in our body are in the abdomen, near the location of the second chakra, which is where Eastern tradition puts the sex drive. Therefore, attitudes toward sex do play into both of those lower chakras for Americans.

As Americans, we get sex thrown at us from the day we are born in the form of media. Sex sells everything. You can see sexualized people on TV and billboards, selling everything from cars to liquor. We think about sex more often than we ever actually have sex. Our attitudes are not the same as ancient Tantrics.

What I'm presenting here is a more Westernized chakra layout. Do check other sources, and use what works best for you. There are millions of internet sites, and hundreds of books available on chakras.

The Chakras Explained:

Any place in the body where two energy pathways come into contact with each other, there's a chakra. That means every joint, every point where muscles or cartilage diverges into bone has one. However, you don't have to know them all unless you plan to become a professional acupuncturist. This book focuses on seven main chakras.

Chakras work together with instinctual energies to give human beings our emotions. If you stop and think about where you feel most of the emotion related to each instinct, you begin to understand the chakras. (i.e. "a fear in the pit of my stomach," "all choked up with sadness," "I love you with all my heart".) Emotion is simply Energy in Motion, or E+motion.

It takes intense emotion to block of any of the instinctual energy. When a kid experiences intense emotions while learning how the world works, he begins to tie up his instinctual reactions. These chakras may stay tied up in knots for years. It is the student's job to unravel each.

Below is a general outline of the chakras. Each one will vary with individuality, so don't take it as an absolute. However, you may find your individual research and meditations give a deeper understanding of the other aspects of each chakra. Many books in the bibliography go over the chakras much more in depth, but for this course of study, this works well.

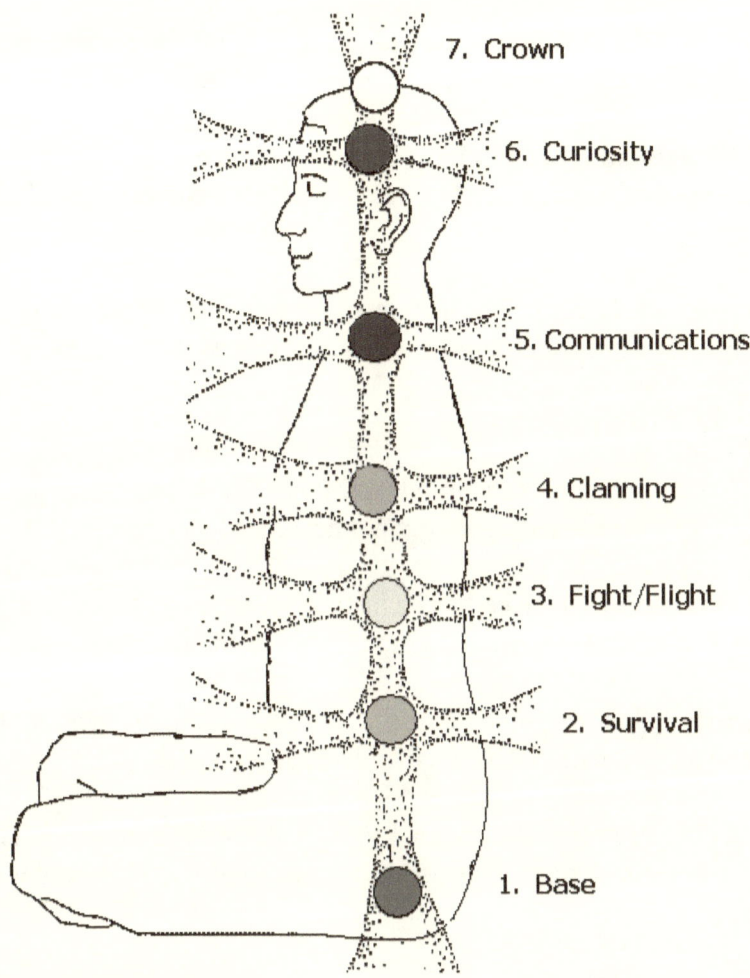

Lower Chakras:

We share these instincts with most animals. Because it takes intense emotional experiences to impact instinctual energy and tie up certain chakras, intense environments train children to ignore or obsess on certain instincts, and therefore create problems with their chakras.

†**Base (1ˢᵗ, Red):** The instinct to perpetuate the species. This includes

major bodily functions and personal survival. Violent abuse victims typically have issues with this chakra.

†**Survival (2ⁿᵈ, Orange):** The instinct to care for the physical body. This includes affection as well as food/water/sleep.

Fight/Flight (3ʳᵈ, Yellow): The instinctual reaction to danger. Situations that require quick thought are impaired with this chakra blocked.

Clanning (4ᵗʰ, Green): The instinct to create bonds of love with other humans. Dysfunctional families tend to tie knots in this chakra

Higher Chakras:

These are the instincts unique to higher life forms. Some people have these chakras activated, but not necessarily all people.

Communication (5ᵗʰ, Blue): The instinct to share one's thoughts and ideas. This includes written communications and gestures.

Curiosity (6ᵗʰ, Indigo): The instinct to know more, to seek out the unknown. This includes science and art, as well as gossip.

Spirit (7ᵗʰ, Violet): The instinct to seek out a higher power. This chakra is usually open in students of metaphysics, philosophy, or spirituality.

(†The influence of these two chakras is typically reversed between Western and Eastern mindsets and cultures. Both chakras are involved in Sexuality. We present here a balanced viewpoint.)

Exercise: Flower Bud Meditation:

This meditation works best if one is already familiar with the chakras. It includes visualizing a flower that blooms and a light that shines outward. It does not matter what variety of flowers your mind puts into the meditation, nor what color the light, but you should pay attention to how healthy those flowers seem to be, and how bright or steady the light is. Pass over any flower or light that does not react immediately until the end of the meditation, and then revisit it. Equalize the rhythm of the breath and the timing allotted to each chakra.

Begin in a quite, sacred space, either sitting lotus-style on the floor, or standing with both feet planted evenly. Begin Pranayama.

As you inhale, put your attention on your base chakra. Visualize a new, closed flower bud at that location. As you exhale, see the flower bud open and the petals emerge. Inhale again and visualize a beam of light shining directly downward from your base chakra into the ground. As you exhale, relax into the sensation it causes, and move your attention up to the next chakra.

With the next breath, put your attention on your second chakra. Visualize a closed new flower bud at that location. As you exhale, see the flower bud open and the petals emerge. Inhale again and visualize a beam of light shining directly outward from your second chakra into the universe in front of you. As you exhale, relax into the sensation it causes, and move your attention up to the next chakra.

With the next breath, put your attention on the space right below your ribs, the third chakra. Visualize a closed new flower bud at that location. As you exhale, see the flower bud open and the petals emerge. Inhale again and visualize a beam of light shining directly outward from your second chakra into the universe in front of you. As you exhale, relax into the sensation it causes, and move your attention up to the next chakra.

With the next breath, put your attention on your heart chakra. Visualize a closed new flower bud at that location. As you exhale, see the flower bud open and the petals emerge. Inhale again and visualize a beam of light shining directly outward from your heart chakra into the universe in front of you. As you exhale, relax into the sensation it causes, and move your attention up to the next chakra.

With the next breath, put your attention on your throat chakra. Visualize a closed new flower bud at that location. As you exhale, see the flower bud open and the petals emerge. Inhale again and visualize a beam of light shining directly outward from your throat chakra into the universe in front of you. As you exhale, relax into the sensation it causes, and move your attention up to the next chakra.

With the next breath, put your attention on your Sixth chakra, right above your eyes. Visualize a closed new flower bud at that location. As you exhale, see the flower bud open and the petals emerge. Inhale again and visualize a beam of light shining directly outward from your Sixth chakra into the universe in front of you. As you exhale, relax into the sensation it causes, and move your attention up to the next chakra.

With the next breath, put your attention on your Crown chakra. Visualize a closed new flower bud at that location. As you exhale, see the flower bud open and the petals emerge. Inhale again and visualize a beam of light shining directly upward from your Crown chakra into the universe above. As you exhale, relax into the sensation it causes, and move your attention up to the next chakra.

If you had any chakras that did not react appropriately, go back to them now and attempt to get them to open or shine. Don't expend too much energy on the task, but remember which chakras are problematic, and recognize that you'll need to work on these places.

When you have opened them all, go back to each of them and adjust them to comfortable levels of opened or closed, bright or dim. Remember to write down which chakras you needed to pay attention to, because this is information your conscious mind will choose to forget.

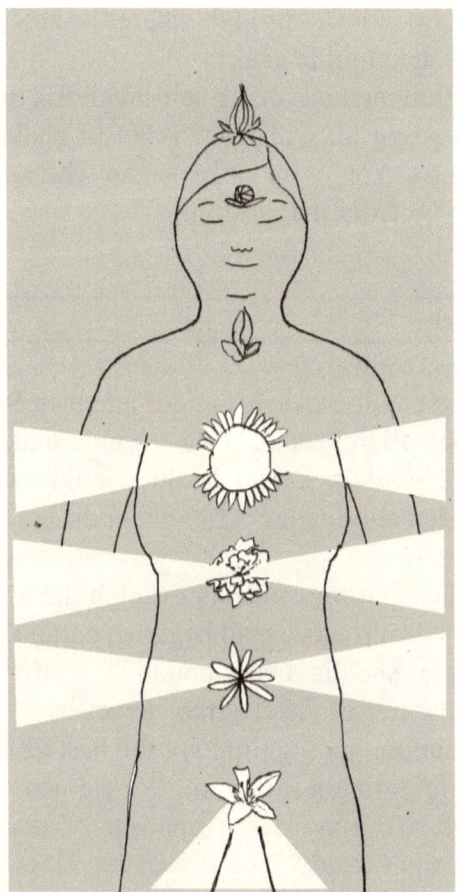

Flower Bud meditation, halfway done

The Flower Bud meditation works very well as a diagnostic tool. If you find a location where you can't see the flower, the flower won't open, or the light won't shine, this would indicate a chakra that needs work. Students who have a hard time with visualizations can imagine skin sensations or musical tones to the same effect.

Many of the issues with chakras are due to the "backpressure" behind it. Energy is supposed to be coming in, moving about, and flowing out. If there's any

> Flower bud: A meditation that becomes a diagnostic tool for chakra blockages.

stoppage, the pressure will build up. It must escape somewhere else. Sometimes it comes out as bad health, bad luck, or both. Usually the escaping energy comes through where the stuck chakra is, in a subject matter related to that chakra.

The Flower Bud meditation is a self-diagnosis tool. How are you feeling? What's going on with you? A lot of chakra work is stuff nobody else can fix. You're the only person who can get inside and see what's going on from that position.

A Giggling Girl:

"R" took my class right around her 30th birthday. She had a bubbly and talkative personality, and contagious laughter. She also suffered from elusive food allergies that at times could make her miserable enough to miss workdays. Her health would roller coaster for months as she tried eliminating different foods, but nothing seemed consistently effective.

During class, I put my students through the above meditation in real time, as a group. As we all began opening the third chakra, R began to giggle. She did a very good job of stifling the laughter as we finished the rest of the chakras, however, when we all came out of the meditation, her giggling got the best of her. The rest of the class began giggling a little too. We calmed down, and then asked what was so funny. Her response: "I don't know, I just can't keep a straight face!" The rest of the class thought THAT was hilarious, and they all began laughing again too. Suddenly, the entire classroom burst into peals of joviality, taking us a few moments to return to the subject of chakras.

Finally, she admitted that any time she focused on the center of her body, she would giggle. She said that she knew she held tension in that area of her body, and was resisting letting it out in tears or anger. We managed to finish the class, but the giggles never entirely went away. Every other student in the class was catching the giggles from R, and it must have been the funniest class ever.

After working with her one-on-one, she discovered that she had held the memory of past sexual molestation in this area of her body. Her internal program said this part needed protecting, so she went out of her way to keep the energy from flowing through that chakra. After working with a therapist and going through different treatments to remove toxins from her system, she was able to pay attention to the center of her torso without it causing giggles. Soon afterward, she found the exact right diet and the food allergies cleared up as well. Eventually, she was able to do the Flowerbud Meditation without giggling.

Projecting Energy: how it works

The thoughts in your head are constantly pushing energy outward from your body in the form of your aura. This is true for everyone. When someone is broadcasting from a particular chakra, even if it's attractive or repulsive, you're going to feel it in the same chakra it came from. You broadcast it like radio frequency. You can tune into it. When you notice someone else's sexual broadcast, you will broadcast your own sexual response without even knowing it. Someone else being hungry will make you hungry. Only those who have intense shielding are protected from the impacts of these energies.

If you're engaged in any way with anyone, exchanging energy, you are performing Tantra. You can have an intellectual, communicative, instinctive, or bonding interaction much the same way we do with sex. This training teaches us how to integrate our experiences and accept all things that come to us.

Energy is just energy right? It's not bad, it's not good, it's just energy. The same electricity that warms hot water will kill a prisoner on death row. You can't judge electricity or energy by what it does and does not do. It's how we use it. Someone's energy coming at you is not good or bad. It just is.

Other People's Chakra Problems

Chakra work teaches us is to change and gauge our chakras so that we can have a controlled impact on the people around us. We can engage—or cease to engage—in other people's energies and actions when we learn to use our own. When you know your chakras independently, you can direct the energy, instead of *being directed by* it.

If you recognize that a person is having chakra issues, you can gauge your chakras accordingly and avoid conflict issues. However, you have to be aware of your own energy to be able to see where other people are coming from.

Figuring out your own chakras makes it easier to get along with people. If they are communicating with you directly from the throat chakra, it's best to communicate with them from there. You train yourself to adjust your own chakras, because it's much easier to control your own chakra pattern than it is to control other people or situations.

On the other hand, recognize also that this is how people react to you, too. Most people just get vibed out with intense broadcasting, but when you learn to gauge your own chakras, you can pheel exactly which chakra that energy is coming from, which gives you a better chance of reacting to it in a positive way.

You'll be able to tell when someone is trying to be artificially friendly, and the social aspect of whether or not someone is truly hitting on you. If they are attempting to make eye contact with you, but you're feeling it at your base, you know something is fishy. You can take advantage of your awareness in all interactive situations.

The more we are aware of it the more pronounced it becomes and the more useful it is to us. Try different combinations and watch other people's reactions to you. Are people really attacking/criticizing/complimenting you? It's useful to be a chameleon in this way, and to adapt yourself to situations instead of expecting the situations to adapt to you.

There are times when a lot of energy is coming in and out of one specific chakra, such as during sex, intense communications, tearful welcomes, traumatic events, and the like. This movement creates a back and forth energy that raises the vibration of the rest of the body. At that point, all the chakras communicate and react on the same level as the highest vibrating chakra.

Connections:
Psychic links that allow one person to be aware of the emotional mindset of another person without the usual clues of verbal or facial expression.

Prisoners of war, people in car accidents together, and those who eat together regularly will create lifetime connections, because their vibrations sync up at the highest level possible. Whatever you are broadcasting is in your control, and that affects everyone around you.

Sexual broadcasting:

Sex is the most obvious form of energy we can exchange. In just about any American nightclub, you find people shooting their energy from the waist down, throwing their hips around on the dance floor, maneuvering through the crowd, more conscious of their butts than their heads. You can tell who walks in to get laid. It's the swagger, it's the flirt, it's the look, and it's the vibe. This is obvious to most people entering the scene. It's primal, it's crass, and it's one of the heaviest hitting forces that we have.

But that's the point of it; you're supposed to notice it. Even if you don't recognize that there's a sex vibe flooding the room, you may have found yourself in a similar crowd starting to have sexual thoughts. Like "Gee, I'm horney tonight" for no reason. It's because you ran in to someone else's base chakra going off...maybe someone who wasn't even attracted to you or attractive to you, but you're feeling the vibe.

Exercise: Gaging other people's reactions to you

When you go out into the world, with your chakras radiating, what does the rest of the world get from you? Do differences in time and mood matter? What about when you are in moments of power? These are important questions to answer if you are to understand your own energy and gain complete control of it.

Why? Your energy level influences your personality. Your environment influences your energy level. Your behavior influences your environment. Your personality influences your behavior.

To break this cycle, you have to break the one element that is totally under your control: your energy. To break that cycle, you must understand what it has been doing while you've not been paying attention all these years.

Take 7 days in a row (one week) and lighting up each chakra for one day out of that week. If you have an ordinary American schedule, you should be able to schedule the days for base and crown on your days off work or school.

By lighting up, I mean adding extra energy to the chakra to keep it open all the time, broadcasting intentionally, within your command. It's easiest to focus on one at a time to begin with. Have that one chakra overly functional, while toning down the other six, and then become observant of the people in your surroundings.

This is an experiment; treat it as such. Keep track as best you can of who reacted how to what chakra. Gather your data at the end of the week and see what you have learned on a larger scale. Chances are, this exercise will not only give you practice in controlling your own energies, it will give you a taste of exactly how powerful Tantric training can be.

A Hearty Hearth

One student, "N," was skeptical about this concept, and went home to try this exercise. What he found blew his mind. He was a blacksmith at a local historic tourist attraction, and spent a whole weekend pounding metal around the hot hearth with only his heart chakra open. About midday, he found his booth surrounded by people who were saying things like "Oh, my grandpa was a blacksmith..." and "Wow, I remember watching that as a kid." He would stop his work and chat with them as often as he could. Almost all of his interactions had something very heartfelt about them. He said he had a blast with the day, but learned that this energy was worth some close attention.

Blockages

What blocks a chakra is fear--fear of something not under your control. Perhaps this block helped you survive a rough time in the past, or perhaps it has been protecting you from certain situations. Either way, it was useful to you at some point, but now it is no longer useful.

This is why you are studying Tantra at all.

The courage and conviction it takes to lay down your fears, to accept and surrender to the Here and Now, even in the face of great adversity, takes a lot of trust in the universe. To understand that sort of trust—that Perfect Trust—takes some way to check the answers to the existential questions that you have to ask.

Who can truly answer the question "Am I doing this right?" Who can truly tell you what career to follow, which book to believe, what teacher to accept? There is only one source. The Naked Flame.

To have clear chakras is to give the Naked Flame permission to interact directly with the Universe, free to make it's Will manifest, and free to point you in the right direction. This may be difficult to grasp now, but when re-reading this book later, you will come to know it for sure.

Exercise: Heart Cave Meditation:

Sit quietly in lotus position on the floor, or upright in a chair. Close your eyes and relax, begin meditative breathing. Visualize yourself sitting inside your own heart.

It should appear as a red-walled cave. However this manifests is how it is supposed to look for now. Get up, explore the walls of the cave, and see if you can see or feel any damage; holes, tears, dirt, rips, anything that seems unhealthy. Repair any holes. If you need any tools, you'll find them laying on the floor. Pull the edges together, smooth over any cracks or tears with your hands. Clean up all dirt, chip off any hard growths, make the walls healthy again.

Go all the way around the cave, including the floor and ceiling. It might take some time. If you can't finish it all in one visit, look at the damage, decide what you need to do, and promise your self to come back and finish the job later. Approach it as you would any long-term project.

Once you have cleaned up the heart to the best of your ability, return to the center of the cave and center and ground yourself. Feel the happiness of a clean environment, and allow yourself to relax in a better feeling place. When you are comfortable sitting there, turn around and look behind you. You should see a person there that looks like you, but with some differences. This is the Inner Self. Make a note of anything that is not identical to how you look here and now in your life. If there is any real injury or pain to this figure, try to help him/her heal.

Give your Inner Self a hug, the kind of hug you would give a loved one who has just returned from a long absence. Feel your bond to this person. Even if you are not a 'visual' type of meditator, you can do most of this work by feel.

Pay close attention to the differences between you and the inner double in this meditation. He/she represents something that your conscious mind has tried to hide; your inner self has clues for you that are not available any other place. Try asking him/her if there is any information that you need to know. Also ask what you can do to make their lives easier, or if there are changes that you could make that would allow you to grow faster. Remember their advice!

When you are done learning all you can from the inner double, thank him or her and promise to return. Let your inner double know how grateful you are that they are there, on the job, doing what they do. Hugs, gifts, and other symbols of gratitude are appropriate. This is a place you should be comfortable visiting, and you should make a point of returning over and over, until you feel that the Inner Self is identical with the Outer Self, and you have totally repaired and cleaned the heart.

Then say good-bye, return to the center of the cave, and sit down again. Slowly bring yourself back to common reality, retaining what you learned from the inner double. Write it down if it's very important. You have just met the best friend you will ever have.

Why is this meditation so effective? Our subconscious mind only has a few different methods of getting through to our conscious mind. Meditation and visualization are the easiest ways for our forebrain and our subconscious mind to communicate. This also allows us a method to self-check what we are learning in books and websites, as well.

American Twilight Language:

In America, we use a type of twilight language in mass media, sexually suggestive if only you know the code. In the 70's, AC/DC came out with a song called "The Jack," which, in the recorded version had references to meeting a woman, but also to a game of cards. In the live version, Angus Young asks his audience to yell back the word "clap" rather than "Jack", which in itself is also twilight language, slang for a sexually transmitted disease. This gave the song yet another meaning.

What you find when you unravel the twilight language of Tantra is many different layers, overlying a base of sexual innuendo. While a song such as "The Jack" has only a

> Twilight language:
> Metaphor and double-entendres designed to mask and veil the true meaning of a phrase.

few meanings twilight language has dozens of possible meanings. So, where can you turn to for the best translation of the texts? How can you decipher if "brought to realization of the truth," means that someone was spiritually enlightened, driven from the territory, blissed-out in orgasm, or given the lecture of a lifetime?

The best source for that information is within you. The Inner

> Heart cave:
> A meditation that becomes a diagnostic tool for chakra clearing.

Double that you met in the Heart Cave will give you the meaning you need from the texts as you read them. Other students on the path may have input you need as well. It is a very effective way of learning, however, you must also be willing to tackle the puzzles presented to you by your inner self.

> ### "Too much, Too Little"
>
> A friend, "D", who was a traveling tavern musician as an occupation, had a girlfriend, "N", who stayed home while he was out of town. Both of them came to see me to help patch up their stormy relationship. Walking them both through the heart cave meditation separately was revealing. D's heart was full of brackish water, with cigarette butt and whiskey bottles floating around his ankles in the dark. N's heart, on the other hand, had no walls, only stringy webs to mark where the walls should have been, as if this heart had been bombed in a war. If D had poured the contents of his heart into N, her heart would have let it all flow out again anyway. If N had tried to help drain the mess in D's heart, she would have had no tools to do so.
>
> As they cleaned up their prospective messes internally, they also recognized that there were major differences in life philosophies between them. They separated amicably, and now hold distant-but-friendly conversations. D is now in a satisfying relationship, and N is very much a woman of her own power.

Acceptance/Surrender

All things happen for a reason, all interactions have their place in your life. You may not be happy with the situation, but recognize your satisfaction or dissatisfaction with events is entirely up to you. No one can "make" you feel something. Nobody has gotten into your head to push a lever, and there's no little angry person inside you painting your eyeballs red; it's all your own programming.

The only true pain is the pain of resistance. There is nothing that can hurt the Naked Flame. The body, the mind, the ego, all of that can die, and the Naked Flame will survive.

Fear is all there is between your Naked Flame and your experiences. Fear is useful when we are trying to survive, but we are no longer living in a hunter-gatherer society. Like modern transportation and birth control issues, we can learn to overcome our natural tendencies for the good of the population. We can overcome our primal fears just as easily as we overcame fear of heights, flying, and snakes.

Spiritual Surrender is the term we use to define that point where you lay down all egos, remove all shields and set your Naked Flame free to do what it must do at that moment. When we give up all fear, we see each other for our true selves, which creates an open flow of energy between us. Allow whatever is manifesting to manifest without acceptance or rejection, without suppression or cultivation, whether it comes from another human or some other part of our reality.

To the Naked Flame, Good and Bad are all in the mind. Humans have to decide that everything must be categorized into "like" and "dislike," and then we title those categories "good " and "bad." Even pain can be good, if it means you will be healing soon. Ask a tattoo artist.

> Resistance:
> An intentional stopping of the flow of energy, due to fear or desire. The opposite of Surrender.

Resistance to pain comes from fear of pain. Pain is a part of the human condition, and if the Naked Flame is to have The Complete Human Experience, it must experience human pain. Therefore, pain is not only something to tolerate, but it is something that is necessary to embrace.

If something looks like it's a negative experience, we will resist it with all we got. Any time we are faced with breaking up with someone, telling our boss that we quit, or complaining to someone about his or her behavior, we are looking down the barrel of fear. All of these things are negative experiences that we will resist.

We will put off going to the boss about a coworker's buggy behavior because it's a negative experience. However, to be open to ALL experiences is part of being human. There is no good and bad, there is no positive and negative. There are experiences that will enhance our growth or that will stifle our growth. There is behavior that is adaptive or maladaptive. Nothing more, nothing less.

> Surrender:
> An intentional relaxation that allows any energy flow to continue on its intended course. Surrender is the opposite of Resistance.

To recognize which experience you are in the middle of, you have to be here now, not thinking back to last week or ahead to next week. Be here now, even if you're going to do something that you've been resisting doing. It's like cleaning out closets. We look at them and close the door. That isn't helping to clean the closets.

Exercise: Sexual surrendering

The next time you are in a sexual situation, either with yourself or your partner, relax into the feeling entirely. Give up any thoughts of "this feels good" or "this feels bad". Go with the flow, and surrender yourself to what is happening. Feel every touch you or your lover makes on your body. Allow yourself to be absorbed in the moment.

This also works for painful experiences. The next time you must experience pain, calm yourself down and explain to your Naked Flame, "This is the experience of pain. Embrace it. Allow myself to experience it fully so I don't have to repeat it."

Your mind will begin to gather different perspectives on the pain, and eventually, you find a solution to it buried in one of these new perspectives. Possible untried treatments, or new ways of getting through the pain, become apparent and allow you to clear up the chakra block where the pain originated.

What good is the Ego?

The Ego, all by itself, turns out to be some sort of support network for The Naked Flame. It divides the One Divine Force into different components called "people." It is there to help our Naked Flame get fundamentally set in habits and structures of our environment until we can become mature humans. It is a place to hang our fears, so that the Naked Flame is motivated in a particular direction for that body. We need it to interface with other humans, who are both mature and immature. It gives a foundation that includes our individual personhood, so that other people can communicate with us.

The ego is based in the chakras, and how we have programmed them over the years. Yes, we could, in theory, all live ego-less lives, if we did not have to start off as immature children learning how to function in this world brand new every time. Or if we all matured at the same rate. Or if we all recognized the One Divinity that is in All of us. But, since it's a mixed bag, we all have to deal with the ego as part of the package.

Communication happens thru Ego; otherwise, you have no language, no socialization processes, no peer groups, and no reason for any of it. The Flame can function alone for a short time (when you're dreaming, or in higher meditations). However, when you recognize what the ego actually does for you, you achieve the power to CHANGE it. At Will. Without permission from anyone else.

Surrender to that idea that you are human and shit happens, that everything has a reason for existence. Even if that reason is merely to take up space. Everything that exists will affect the outcome of tomorrow.

When you surrender to that concept and you stop resisting two things happen: First, the negative things come and go real fast. When we finally get off our butt and clean out the closet, we think, "that wasn't so bad. Why was I resisting that?" Second, this puts it behind us, so that it's gone. It no longer clogs up our energy, and it no longer influences our ego. Surrendering to the moment allows us to unplug our ego right here and now.

A popular way of putting that is "to go with the flow." All of these things are basically just energy running thru us. Our experiences are truly just energy coming in and going out. If we resist an experience, it only builds up and mounts pressure against you.

It's very similar to a river dam. The more water you hold back, the bigger the dam has to be, because of the amount of water. When you stop listening to the clues of your Naked Flame, the larger hints get louder and louder, inserting themselves into your daily consciousness, until pretty soon you get whacked in the head with what my mother always called a "clue-by-four." If you ignore your problems long enough, they don't go away; they build up and take you out. This goes for any problem, like paying bills, dealing with health issues, or being hungry.

At some point, the situation becomes a crisis and an emergency. You have to deal with all of it right now. If you allow those situations to come and go all the time, go with the flow and allow yourself to experience whatever it is and learn from it, you 're less likely to have to have that experience again.

This is an often-quoted passage, but every time I read it, it reminds me of what I need to remember. I put it here because of its implications for untying chakras.

"Our deepest fear is not that we are inadequate. Our deepest fear is that we are powerful beyond measure. It is our light, not our darkness, that most frightens us. We ask ourselves, who am I to be brilliant, gorgeous, talented, and fabulous? Actually, who are you not to be? You are a child of God. Your playing small doesn't serve the world. There's nothing enlightened about shrinking so that other people won't feel insecure around you. We are all meant to shine, as children do. We are born to make manifest the glory of God that is within us. It's not just in some of us, it's in everyone. And as we let our own light shine, we unconsciously give other people permission to do the same. As we are liberated from our own fear, our presence automatically liberates others."

--Marianne Williamson
A Return To Love: Reflections on the Principles of A Course in Miracles,
Harper Collins, 1992.
From Chapter 7, Section 3 (Pg. 190-191).

When we mature, we no longer need the ego as a support network, but many of us use it to dim down the Naked Flame, to be less powerful than we are capable of being. We allow it to clog up the chakra mechanisms with fears and old habits, hanging on to the past in a subliminal way.

That works just fine for anyone who doesn't want to study Tantra. Since your job is to increase your vibratory rate to the highest level possible, you don't want to dim down anything anywhere. Let go of all of those constructs that have the label "I am." You are none of that, and much much more.

Groundwork:

White: Flower bud meditation daily for one week. Pay close attention

46

to the flashes of memory that run through your mind as you open and work on each chakra. By the end of the week, you should see some improvement on at least one of the impacted chakras. If you do not, continue the daily Flower bud meditations as you work the further exercises in this book, until you see improvement on at least one chakra.

Red: Couples Karezza: Pick one person to meditate, one person to help. Have the meditator lay nude, totally relaxed, while the helper touches, pets, licks, and/or sexually stimulates the meditator. Allow this mindset to last at least 28 minutes before orgasm. Switch roles the next time. See what effect this has on your chakra connections over time.

Blue: Gauging reactions: Light up a different chakra every day, and see what reactions around you change within the community and in other environments. Take 7 days and keep track of everyone's experiences. Share these as a group, to give everyone a full sense of the purpose of each chakra.

Chapter 3:   The Abyss Ritual

The Abyss is Subconscious

When we first started teaching this class, the exercises in the chapter marked #4 came before those in the chapter marked #3. This is because the Kundalini exercise and the Abyss ritual go together. A former student calls the Abyss Ritual "Cosmic Drain-o" because it allows the Kundalini to flow smoothly through the chakras. It helps you clear your chakras so that you can successfully channel healthy energy.

What is the Abyss? It is the "dark self." It is that black box in the back of your head where you put things you don't want to think about. It is the backpack where you keep all of your psychological baggage. Your fears are there, as well as your secret desires--it's

> Abyss:
> The dark place in the back of our minds where we keep all the things we don't want other people to know about us, or the things we don't want in our thoughts.

your subconscious. The Abyss ritual clears the Abyss.

The subconscious, for the most part, controls what the aura does and how it reacts. Usually it does it's thing without us having to pay attention to it. When someone has an emotional impact like a trauma, it freezes a particular thinking pattern into your nervous system, which includes your brain, spine, and peripheral nerves. This leads to a physical body-based memory that hooks together with the mental and emotional effects of the trauma.

Once a person has had this thinking pattern frozen into their nervous system, all situations that might even come close to that trauma, serve to activate the traumatized thinking pattern, which then activates the body memory, creating the same reaction in your body and brain. It "reactivates" the fear response.

Most people will activate the same fear response over and over in the face of the same triggers, getting the same results. Fear slows down all energetic vibration like cholesterol in a beating heart. Openness to connection (ok, let's call it "love") clears out the channels and speeds up the velocity of energy in the system. It allows your chakras to function correctly.

If a person can control the fear patterns in his or her energy, then the reaction to fearful situations is intuitive, smooth, and without hesitation, looking at all options immediately, and making the right choice with ease. This is the result of a smooth flow of energy through clear channels. We have all had "golden moments" of catching falling items, near-miss driving, speaking the right thing at the right time, and the like. This ability comes from that smooth, no-fear, intuitive energy, what Malcolm Gladwell calls the "thin slice" of thoughts in a flash second. (see bibliography, "Blink")

If the human is filled with fear, or the activation of an old trauma that creates fear, he or she will hesitate before moving during any crisis, making poor decisions and usually making the crisis worse. Such a person typically sees the world in black and white absolutes, especially at that moment of indecision.

When two auras go walking, the loud one does the talking:

Two auras meet when the energies of the two people reach out toward each other, as in conversation, shaking hands, hugging, etc. When this happens, they exchange some personal energy. One person may walk away with more energy, or with less. Auras can also accidentally meet, as in crowded situations, accidental traumas, or going through intense situations together. If one person is in a negative headspace, his/her aura usually brings with it a negative feel, known as psychological baggage, which can be contagious. This negative feel can be passed from one person to another, such as with a complaining friend who brings you down after each conversation.

When two auras meet, there is usually a kinestetic reaction akin to static electricity or sound-wave vibrations between the two people. This is an exchange of subtle communication between two people. This very muted, mild skin sensation is transferred to the brain through your nerves. Once it gets there, it sets off quick memories associated with the current situation. Your energies shift to be more in line with the other person, for better communications. Since the aura is controlled by your own subconscious thoughts, it's usually adjusted by the subconscious part of the brain; the same part responsible for bringing you the heartbeat and the breathing rate.

When you do Pranayama breathing as in Lesson 1, you attack this automatic adjustment system from the other side; you take over the subconscious work of breathing and heart rate. This will allow the subconsicous to be up front and show you what it has been doing with your energy all this time while you weren't looking.

Socialization vs. instincts

The most difficult thing Americans have to deal with when learning Tantra is dropping the paradigm of American sexuality. American culture socializes people to view sex as bad, dirty, and wrong. We see sex used as a weapon, a lure, a trap, and a prize. Our media is filled with images of what we are led to believe is "desirable" sexuality, but it doesn't look like the real people we see. They tease us, and then chastise us to abstain.

Sex is just another instinct, like eating, sleeping, and playing. We are mammals; mammals have penises and vaginas, and they have sexual intercourse. Since sex is something we cannot get away from, (like food and sleep) we have the responsibility for enabling that instinct in a socially acceptable manner. There are social norms that surround food and sleep, rules that we all follow or risk being embarrassed, like falling asleep in class or eating in a sloppy fashion. As such, sex has its rules too.

However, we are just beginning to understand the rules around civilized sex. Why? Because for many years, sex was a taboo subject, not fit for discussion in public. In the last 50 years, the taboos surrounding sex have been falling by the wayside in light of scientific discovery and an equalization of genders. This makes Tantra very necessary for the healing of American sexuality.

To open up to Tantra is to forget all of your former prejudices about sex, whether prudish or liberal. When you forget the things that you once believed to be true about sex, you can begin experiencing it in the here and now. If you are relaxed and focusing only on the feelings of the present, giving it 100% of your attention, you'll get 100% of the experience. No looking at the future (toward the orgasm) or thinking about the past (allowing baggage to come up). Just be here and now. It's like anything else in life; to do the best job possible, you need to take your time.

Tasting Energy:

Every time two auras meet, there is an exchange of energy. However, we tend to keep those interactions on the surface of our auras, not allowing them to affect us deeply. Very rarely does the Naked Flame of one person ever contact the Naked Flame of another person. There are so many layers between people, the Naked Flame can only observe, as if from behind heavy glass.

To remove that barrier means to unblock the chakras, face down fears and deal with hidden desires. Once we have done all of that, the aura allows other people's energy to get closer, but it still does not go all the way. To contact the Naked Flame, we need to make it happen. All shields—and I mean all—need to come down. Only sex can do that. The allure of sexual contact with this much closeness is exactly what makes Tantra enticing in the first place.

Many people make that happen by accident with intense sex. A lot of times it happens unintentionally, as a side effect from long-term contact with another person, or living through a traumatic event with someone. All of these situations allow us (or force us) to drop our shields. To intentionally connect your Naked Flame to another person's Naked Flame is a cornerstone of Red (or partnered) Tantra, and a skill you must cultivate before going into higher rites. One can practice this ability with the following exercises:

Exercise: Opening Up:

Pick someone you are close to, someone who may know your deepest darkest secrets. (This is listed as a Red Tantra groundwork exercise). You don't have to verbalize these secrets, however, you must find yourself comfortable with the prospect of this person learning every bit of information about you, public and private. If you have no one like this in your life, do not attempt this exercise, but go on to the Abyss meditation and find out why you have no one this close to you.

Now, engage this person in a face-to-face conversation, with no table, desk, counter, or other furnishings between you. It doesn't matter what you discuss, but something with emotional content works best. As you listen to this individual, drop all of the outer layers of energy you can visualize. Imagine your friend seeing all the way into you, as you absorb the words they are saying. As soon as you have opened up all of your defenses, you should be able to psychically 'pheel' which chakra(s) your friend is broadcasting from, and even possibly what emotion your friend is broadcasting. Some describe it as a tickle, some describe it as a temperature change, but you will find one chakra being "activated." Your first impression is usually the most accurate.

You need only do this for one moment to get a taste of the energy coming at you. I don't recommend doing it much longer than that, because it quickly creates connections between people that may or may not need to be there. Hopefully, you will attempt the exercise with this in mind, and choose your partners wisely.

When you have taken a piece of their energy into your system, visualize your own energy to see where you pheel it the strongest. Chances are, this chakra is the one they are broadcasting from. Put that information together with the content of their words and the expression on their face, and see how close all three match up. The more honest someone is, the clearer their chakras are, and the most consistently matching their chakras, expressions, and stories will be.

Your Own Personal Jesus:

You can also view Tantra as a religion. Many philosophers have tried to discover exactly why human beings need religion. This question would never be asked if not for our need for consensus reality. If you have been Christian, Jewish, or Islamic, you may know the security that comes in having faith in an energy source larger than your self. However, most Americans, even those raised in patriarchal faiths, have come to see God in a different light than our ancestors. "He" is no longer a solid figure sitting on clouds; "He" is now an abstract energetic concept that somehow caused the Big Bang and everything after it.

The Americans who look to other systems such as Tantra for

answers to life's questions are usually not the same type of person to blindly hang hope upon a vague and abstract concept. As it says in the song by Depeche Mode, we all need someone to hear our prayers, someone who cares. We all need to think that in the darkest of moments that someone somewhere loves us.

In Tantra, we name our "God" Shiva and our "Goddess" Shakti.

> Shakti:
> the Feminine aspect of Divinity.

These are not people-oriented Deities as we know Deities in the West. These are concepts like Einstein's Mass and Energy: they exist everywhere in everything and they have a job to do.

If you are not one to hang your spirituality on Deities created from someone else's fantasy, you may try considering the Deities as specific principles that are within

> Shiva:
> the Masculine aspect of Divinity

other humans, such as the spark of life, or the energy in our cells. Considering what Shiva stands for, you can also create your own construct of who/what he is. Shiva is depicted traditionally blue to associate him with the sky. Shakti's skin is the color of sand or soil, because she is a symbol of the Earth. When they come together, sky and earth, they create everything we know. Earth and Sky together make our environment possible. The sacred female, the sacred male. The Omnipotent Orgasm between Shiva and Shakti is recreated every time that you orgasm with your lover.

You can also equate Shiva with Einsteins "matter" and Shakti with his "Energy" in the $E=MC^2$ equation. Neither Shiva nor Shakti is a "god" as western Americans learn "god." They are forces more akin to gravity than to any patriarchal God. It's a natural law. There really are no personalities to them, there's just a force that is masculine and a force that is feminine.

Doing research and finding your favorite Deities, or making your own up if you need to, is possible, because it's not about the personality of a Deity. Worshipping in Tantra is about receiving those energies of Shiva and Shakti, above and below, masculine and feminine. It's not about what you call them or how they look, it's about opening up to those forces and bringing them into yourself, then creating an outward moving wave for your environment to change as well.

Mandalas, Malas, Yogas, Yantras, Mantras, Mudras, and Other Mystic Stuff:

Different types of sacred arts and objects have always inspired eastern thought. The earliest known art in the world, east or west, was for religious purposes. No one in America can think about Buddhism without thinking of the delicate sculptures and giant paintings that accompany all Buddhist ritual. These items help students stay focused, especially in traditional teaching relationships.

There are some traditions that work well in creating the environment to help the headspace you need. Some of these items require thoughtful purchase or creation. The bibliography may help the curious reader. The following is only a limited list of the most commonly used methods, and a brief overview of each one.

Mandalas: A Mandala is a symmetrical picture made of interlocking shapes and small pictures that create a meditative pattern. It always begins with a central point, and typically has four balanced quarters, and have been printed and published on everything from temple walls to coffee mugs. Making the mandala, they say, is the meditation itself. The giant sand paintings of the Tibetan monks are examples of Mandala meditations.

Mala: A mala is a string of prayer beads, like a rosary, but they are not for praying, they are for chanting. All malas utilize the sacred numbers of 12 and 9. There are usually 109 beads on a mala (12 X 9 + 1 "guru bead"), and the purpose is to allow you to do repetitions of mantras without having to count them all.

Yoga: This typically means "union" in its purest translation, but then again, the rest of these terms can be considered Yogas as well. In America, what we consider Yoga is actually Hatha Yoga, a method of movement and poses that creates a meditative state. "Hatha Yoga" or "Mudra yoga" includes more than the described motion--they also include concentration and focus on that motion to the point of deeper understanding of the physical or energetic body. If you practice yoga, realize that there's nothing "perfect" in the poses themselves; mental concentration on your body muscles creates the meditative headspace.

Yantras: A Yantra is a sacred symbol, or a two dimensional picture usually created for a specific purpose that is universal, such as to one specific deity. Yantras need not be symmetrical, nor symbolic; some Yantras are actual pictured Deities. Many yantras, such as the famous "Sri Yantra" are also Mandalas, but not all Mandalas are Yantras.

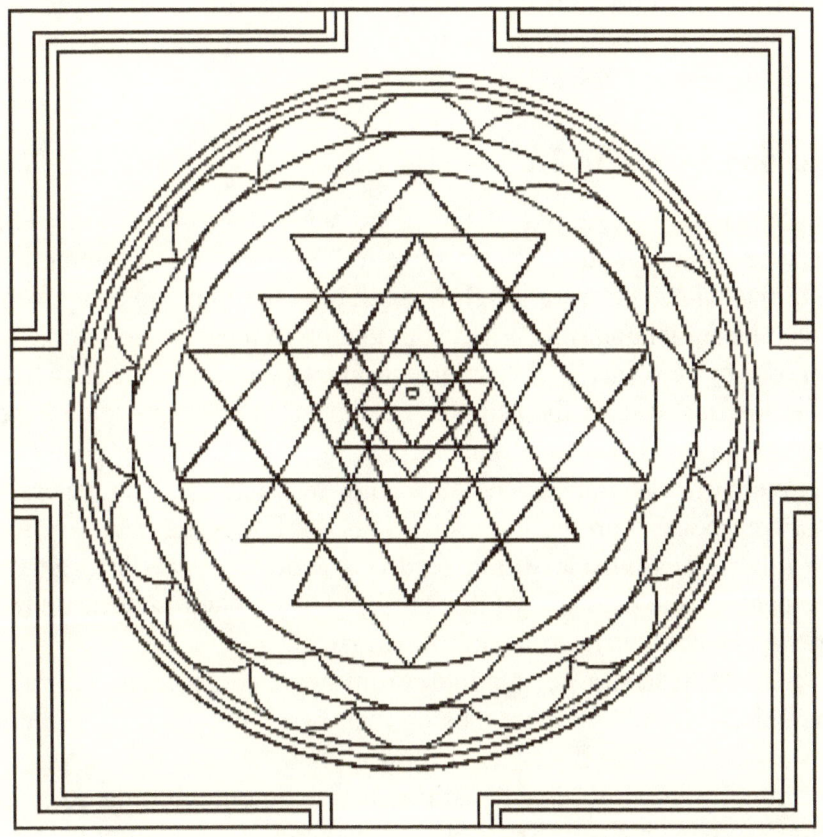

The Sri Yantra, a symbol of Shakti, is also a mandala

Mantras: A mantra is a sound—usually a series of syllables—verbalized repeatedly until it becomes the background noise to the meditation. Traditionally, a guru will give you a mantra. Mantras are typically specific to a purpose, such as invoking or thanking particular deities.

Mudras: These are simply hand or body gestures that usually

align several of the 144,000 chakras in the body somehow, so that your meditation includes certain circuits. Holding the middle finger and thumb together above the palm of the hand is a common mudra to help open the palm chakra. Again, mudra forms are a yoga that requires pointed attention, not just going through the motions.

By utilizing these methods and items, the ancients created shortcuts and environments that helped them on their paths. You don't need to know all these things to make Tantra work for you, however, if you want to study the depth of this path, I recommend studying any of these subjects in detail.

Getting Down To It:

What does the Abyss have to do with chakra clearing? The nervous system is just that—a system. It's a network of interacting neurons, whose information flows both too the brain and away from it via the spinal column. When you hold on to fears in the brain, the nervous system carries this information into the rest of the network. The nervous system then tightens up muscles, effects organs, and creates physical postures that keep energy from flowing correctly thorough our system. This posture sends messages back to the brain that your body is protecting itself. This reinforces the fear. To clear up this nerves-muscles-brain feedback loop, one needs to get to the heart of the psychology that created the problem to clear up the energy. Hence, the need for the Abyss ritual.

People in health occupations, from heart surgeons to massage therapists, will tell you that they do their best work when the patient has a mental leap in their own healing as well. Modern psychologists are now teaching about a "brain/body" dichotomy, but the ancient Tantrics knew this as a "Tri-chotomy": Brain, Body, and Energy. This is why there are usually 3 different aspects of any given concept in Hindu Pantheon. Shiva: Vishnu, Brahma, Krishna. Shakti: Parvati, Laxmi, Kali.

> Tri-chotomy:
> The connection of Mind, Body, and Spirit.

When applied to your own healing, if you correct one of the 3, the other 2 will adjust themselves. Fix the body and the psychology and energy will self-correct. Fix the psychology and the body and energy will self-correct. Fix the energy, and you see the same pattern emerge. The Abyss works on the energy, but uses the body and the psychology to get there.

Clues:

Pranayama takes us into higher mental functions that normal breathing cannot. To attain these higher functions is to self-correct your energy—to put it where it's supposed to be, as opposed to what is making it unhealthy and unable to flow. Each time we succeed at an exercise, we self-correct and heal.

There are several different ways to fix one's chakra problems. You can raise your vibration to a higher level and allow the unhealthy energies to shake out. You can address unhealthy thought patterns by asking, "What makes me carry this fear?" and therefore unravel the psychology behind it. You can have a health professional help straighten out any muscular or organic dis-ease. All of these lead you to the same result: clear chakras and healthier energy.

When you come to the point of raising Kundalini later in your studies, it will not function correctly if any of your chakras have lingering baggage, . You can find yourself radiating energy from a point that is not under your conscious control. This, of course, will cause you to manifest the situations that you fear the most. For example, if you have a fear of speaking out, your throat chakra is probably blocked. When you elevate your energy in any way, you will find a need to speak out, day after day, until you learn to drop that fear. Sometimes those lessons can be quite harsh.

The best solution is to catch your fears before you attempt to raise a large amount of energy such as the Kundalini exercise in the next chapter. However, it may be helpful to use both Abyss ritual and Kundalini meditation, in tandem, to work through your chakras one by one in successive fashion. Exposing your chakra knots is the hard part, the part only you can do. The next chapter goes into the relationship of the Abyss to Kundalini in more detail.

Exercise: Abyss Ritual

Once your Chakra knots are exposed, and you know what sort of problem you are working on, you can begin untying them. If you find they take up too much of your headspace don't hesitate to perform this exercise.

Set aside several hours where you can be undisturbed in temple space. Light your favorite incense and candles to remind your self this is a magickal act. Create your sacred temple space around the entire room, so that you have as much freedom of movement as possible.

Now, just sit back and think about your past. Think about your parents, siblings, and friends growing up. Start thinking about the chakra you are working on, and what may have caused that block. You may know this right off the top of your head; if this is the case, it is probably something you have avoided thinking about for a long time. Now, you MUST think about it. This is the purpose of this ritual.

If the memory isn't apparent, think about your block. Put the impact of your greatest fear into motion by imagining a scenario that would invoke it. (For example, if you're greatest fear is loneliness, imagine yourself stranded in a strange place.)

Name that emotion. Put a handle on it. Now, ask yourself "When was the first time I felt this emotion?" If you can't remember the first time, try to find the earliest occurrence of this emotion in your life. Somewhere in your past you made an emotion-based decision that "The world works this way." This decision is wrong for you because it is contrary to your Naked Flame. However, it sticks in your inner programming, confusing your entire being, and causing knots in your psyche.

Once you remember the very __first__ time you felt this emotion, replay the scene in your head with as much detail as you can remember. Think about the location, the people present, the furniture or weather that day. Figure out all the details and relive the scene in your mind as vividly as possible. Put yourself firmly in that reality.

As soon as you can pheel the emotion-laden energy begin to rise in yourself (tears, anger, shame) begin the Karezza exercise. This may be difficult at first, but it might help to visualize the emotion draining out of your system into the ground. You might find it flowing outward with the Karezza-generated waves of energy.

Let go of that energy as you relive the scene in retrospect. Keep your physical body distracted by your hand, and remember you can separate physical from emotional here. You are letting go of the emotional by keeping the physical body occupied with something very pleasant.

Some questions to think about are:

How old were you when that chakra was first impacted?
Where were you? Describe the room and any objects you see.
Who else is there?
What is happening?
What is being said?
What are you feeling?
What would you like to say or do?

Sometimes, at this point, you need is to say what it was you didn't say in the past. Scream it if necessary. Get it out there! Pour it out anyway it wants to come. Don't stop it just because it is uncomfortable. Remember, you are in a safe, secure, sacred space you created yourself. There's no sense in you stuffing that emotion again. Cry, yell, or fall apart emotionally, BUT KEEP UP THE KAREZZA until you have made it over the cliff and into orgasm. Then float in that space for the rest of this exercise.

You may find hidden memories. Do not back down from these memories! You must do this with perfect love and perfect trust in yourself. This moment is a very volatile one for you. You may need to rely on you own intuitions to know exactly what to do. Use your instinct and pheelings to get through it. When the bulk of emotional energy is gone, keep floating. Ask yourself what conclusions the "younger you" came to at that time. You must find the fault in this thinking yourself. Is the "younger you" correct in making decisions for the "now you" body? Re-think that decision, and come up with one that applies to your current reality.

Go into the scene again as an observer in your "now you" body. Talk to the "younger you" and all the people involved. Correct the situation in your memory as only a wiser person could. Whether you picture yourself striking your oppressors, or merely speaking to

59

them, you may need to purge more emotional energy at this point as your life lessons flash in your head. You may remember all the times you reacted badly to the same sort of situation. You may find another problem life-lesson now. If so, repeat the process of purging and re-evaluating. Ground the energy as before, until it is all out. You may still find "bubbles" of this energy in the coming days; ground it out whenever you find it.

Know that the scene will never happen again, and no one will ever be able to push those buttons in you again. Ground out any residual energy and clean up your sacred space. Sleep immediately after you do this rite! You will probably be exhausted anyway. Your subconscious mind must sort through this stuff before your conscious mind.

When you wake up, you should feel rested and light.

You will float for several days after this as the puzzle pieces of your psyche rearrange themselves. Floating feels like being inside a large pillow, or seeing life through a fog. It is an instinctive reaction to untying knots and should not scare you. (Some students say they feel high. Enjoy it.) Try to keep yourself from spending these days in solitude. At this point, anything offered to your brain as "truth" will either be accepted or rejected without question, so be careful where you go and who you talk to.

If you seem to feel normal, without floating, it could be you haven't purged enough energy from the knot. As you have come this far, and your decision was rectified, you will slowly leak the energy out on your own. Keep an eye on your old behavior patterns, (which won't go away as easily) and ground any emotional energy you feel attached to them. The whole purpose of your learning Tantra is to become best person you can be. This means changing the old behavior patterns into something you would rather have.

If you are still floating a week later, you have more knots to untie. Do the exercise again while you are still floating, but change some aspect of it (the temple space, the lighting, or the background sounds) so that you can remember the two rituals as separate events. Your memory of this time will be splotchy, so keep writing in your journal every day. In the event that you know there are several knots to untie, you may take them all apart in one day, but this becomes hard work.

You should not try to do anything overly energetic until you are solidly back on your feet and not floating any longer. You will see the world in a whole new light after this, and any natural obstacles will be easy to remove.

You may choose to have a friend or mentor help you with this ritual by prompting you with the questions and giving you feedback on your answers. If you choose to take that direction, make sure you pick someone to help who you can trust with your most intimate secrets, or the ritual will not work.

Numbered Steps of the Tantric Abyss ritual

1. *Find whichever chakra holds the knot. Do this before you enter sacred space.*

2. *Do this ritual nude. Create sacred space where you can lay comfortably.*

3. *Begin Karezza. Make sure you have some raised vibration before going on.*

4. *Look into the memory banks to see where knot came from. Use body memory if you can.*

5. *Relive the experience in imagination.*

6. *Use Karezza generated orgasm to purge all of the energy & stuffed emotions. Allow your instinct to direct which way the energy should flow out of you.*

7. *Go into the memory and 'fix' it, using current perspective. Realize your growth since the time of this memory. You may need to purge more energy.*

8. *Use this floating/meditative time to rearrange any ideas about yourself that may shift, communicate with your guardian, or astral travel. Allow it to last as long as possible.*

9. *Ground ALL residual energy. Banish or clear out the energy, and close the circle after you are totally grounded.*

10. *Go to sleep, so the unconscious mind works on it first.*

11. *Float for a few days until the mind is settled.*

12. *Go forward with a new outlook.*

Optional: WRITE IT ALL DOWN AFTERWARD!

Blocked Sex Chakras and the Pocket Fantasy:

When students first try the Abyss ritual, they are typically surprised to discover their sexual hang-ups. There are a certain percentage of them that will deny having any sexual hang-ups at first, then after a few weeks of practice, they secretly admit to me that they indeed have discovered some programs embedded in their egos regarding sexuality. Sometimes it's as simple as accepting males and females as equals. Sometimes it's a result of past decisions gone badly, embarrassment or hurt at their first sexual encounter, or even worse, childhood sexual abuse.

How can you tell you have a sexual hang-up? Your pocket fantasy will give you away every time. If you have pocket fantasies that other people may think are not "normal," if you have fantasies that you are afraid to share with anyone else, or fantasies that require you to be sneaky or lie to the people you love, then you can believe you have a hang-up. Fantasies such as cross-dressing, anal sex, oral sex, bondage, Sadism, Masochism, theatrical rape, role playing, multi-partner sex, or public sex are typically fantasies that need to be played out in real life to release the energy behind them. This is why B.D.S.M. 'scenes' have such an impact on the people in them; virtual truckloads of energy get unloaded in those venues.

If you have a pocket fantasy that seems to be a hang up and you can arrange it, try to have your fantasy played out somehow. Find the fetish community in your area, or look on line for people who you might be able to hire to help you. You may need to repeat this process more than once to shed light on the whole picture, and that's okay. You'll recognize how quickly it improves your energy.

The Ego:

The ego is the collection of personality traits that we cling to in order to keep our identities intact. Now that you know that you can manipulate chakras, you also know that you can manipulate your own personality. When we find something that clashes with our energy, we can change our energy and remove the confrontation. To change our energy, we must change our thought patterns, which in turn, changes our personality traits.

Our personality traits are dynamic, changing over time, which makes our ego dynamic. We can change it when necessary, and most of us do change parts of it at some point in our lives. This is called "maturing" or, on the streets, "getting over your shit." But there are certain things in our egos that will refuse to budge under normal circumstances. Positive things in your personality traits, like humor, sensitivity, and intellectual style, typically don't change much over one lifetime.

But this is Tantra. And you knew I wouldn't be bringing it up unless it was not only possible but also desirable to change your ego.

What does the ego do in relation to the Naked Flame? Ego covers the Naked Flame. It makes the Naked Flame safe for human interaction. It helps tone down the brightness. It gives other human beings a place to hang their shortened definitions of who we are, so that they have a point of reference with which to communicate.

The ego is something we self-create, based on our backgrounds. Other metaphysical paths—including many martial arts paths—will tell you that you must destroy the ego and (hopefully) rebuild it. What happens when the ego is gone? There is no personality left. No humor, no anger, no intellect.

Since we know that the ego starts in the chakras, and we know that the chakras are dynamic, what happens when the chakras are totally clear? Does that signal the all-famous "ego death?" Does that mean you become totally undefineable to others around you? Yes.... and no.

Once the chakras are clear, and energy is running at maximum capacity through your system, the entire ego is under your control. You can drop pieces of it, or you can put new pieces on. You can activate your old fears, or you can ignore them. You have your choice of "Action" in any situation, not knee-jerk "re-action." You can open and close chakras, change your behavior when necessary, and become the person you most want to become. When the ego is out of the way, there is nothing else holding you down.

The biggest hurdle most people face when looking at the dissolution of the ego is worrying about how others will be able to interface with your Naked Flame. Will they flip out when you choose to do something different, based on your instinct instead of a habit? Will they say, "I don't know you!" and march out?

Who really cares?

Here's what I mean: If your chakras are clear, then you are always vibrating higher than anything in the room is, unless you happen to be in a room full of Tantrics. But, assuming you are hanging out with average people, you can assume you have the shiniest aura in any crowd. If you are putting out the most energy in any room, then you are not absorbing any energy from anyone else in that crowd unless you intentionally do it for yourself. That translates street-wise into "You don't have to take on any of their shit." That goes for their judgmental attitude as well as any other negativity they have. Not only do you not have to take on their shit, they "get" to take on yours. You will actually RAISE the vibration of any people who vibrate lower.

If they get angry and march out on you, it's because that is what they need to do in response to your energy. You can't tailor your life around other people's judgments and still consider yourself free. You must truly give yourself the space to be free.

Americans say we are free to do as we please, however, we are not. Those who have more power in social situations hold us to social standards via threats, insults, and intimidation. Boys receive bullying. Girls get stifled. If you truly believe you are free, just try walking around naked sometime. Freedom means not worrying about what others say or do or how they react or even if you piss them off. The Naked Flame must have its true freedom to manifest its highest vibration.

Energy travels from the most charged area to the least charged area until there is equilibrium. Car batteries do it; so do humans. Tantra puts this law to the test, over and over.

If you are the highest vibrating thing in the room, then you will find yourself giving energy beyond the call of duty. People will see the Naked Flame and fall in love with it. People will see the wisdom and knowledge that you have to share, and they will ask for it. If you are not constrained by time, give all you have to give. This is why you are there at that particular time and place. Don't worry. Your source is infinite.

"Reprogramming the Sex Instinct"

A graduate of the class related this story:

"After attempting the Abyss Ritual the first time, I thought for sure that I failed it. Surely, with my sexuality in question, my sexual relations in an uproar, and my tendency for premature ejaculation couldn't suddenly be worked out by just one outrageous orgasm! I was proven wrong when I fell rapidly to sleep after the exercise.

I dreamt intensely about all the ghosts from my sexual past, all of them chasing me down from behind. There was no escape, as I ran right into my current sexual partners! As I found myself in amorphous sexual encounters, one turned into another, into another, into yet another. Experiencing again and again all the crassness, emotions, fallouts, the shame and the hurt. I wished only for it to end....for me to wake up!

Then slowly, one partner melded into the other, until the point of an indistinguishable love orgy. I lost the sense of self through all of it, my bodily flesh fell away, and a feeling of burning engulfed all my senses. All the fear and shame literally burned away, leaving only the pure bliss and sacred flames of every sexual partner and experience I'd ever had. The pheeling of eternal bliss and universal connections grew into an orgasmic climax that to this day I have yet to achieve in my Red Tantric practices.

I woke up to a world viewed with new eyes, which would never be the same again. I still search for that ultimate Red Tantric experience, but I will never forget this White Tantric experience."

Groundwork:

<u>White</u>: 28 min Karezza (Masturbatitation described earlier). Practice at least 3 times before moving on to the exercises in the next chapter.

Red: Surrender to your lover: Like the exercise in the last lesson, pick one person to be the meditator, one to be the helper, then switch. Begin by both partners facing each other and mentally walking through the steps of the Flower Bud meditation to open the chakras. Then begin making love, slowly, allowing the chakras to remain open as long as they can. The meditator should simply relax and pay attention to the visions in his/her head while the helper makes love to him/her. As the desire within the meditator's system increases, his/her vibration will raise as well. The meditator should open up to this feeling, allowing all systems to surrender to the manipulations of the helper. Trust is the key to this exercise. Both partners must trust each other to be painless, helpful, and most of all kind.

<u>Blue</u>: Fruit and Flowers exercise (described earlier): Fruit and Flowers for all: Put all the apples, flowers, and chocolate on a tray in the center of the circle. Have everyone describe what he or she is experiencing as they hold—then eat—each item.

Chapter 4:   Kundalini

How Karezza does what it does:

Your body is a conduit of energy that runs from above (Shiva) to below (Shakti) most of the time. This is the God-form energy, the Universal Current, Chi force, whatever you want to call it. In normal human beings, this current runs downward, from top to bottom, unless that person starts intentionally moving energy in specific ways, such as using Yoga, Tantra, or other mystic pathways.

Mystics and Tantrics are NOT normal human beings. We strive to balance that downward force with an upward draw. Other mystic paths do the same thing. Wiccans use Earth energy, the Golden Dawn uses the Middle Pillar meditation, and Shamanic journeys go under the earth. Tantrics bring it up in a method called Kundalini Yoga.

Controlling the energy of Shiva-shakti

Shiva is above and Shakti is below, and the two will always strive to meet. No matter where you put them, Shiva and Shakti never repel from each other. Other energies can get in the way of their meeting, but they still draw each other. There is a lot of extra force created when we have them both in balance, pulling and pushing with equal force. In other words, as you bring in the masculine from above downward to the base chakra, (typical human energy flow) and you simultaneously bring up the feminine energy from below to the crown chakra through meditation, (mystic energy flow) you boost your energy tremendously.

The crown chakra faces straight up: We call this the holy Lotus of Vishnu, or the House of Shiva. The base chakra faces straight down, and connects to the Earth. This is the Seat of Kundalini, or the Lap of Shakti energy. The path of the energy can be through your legs or your tailbone, depending on if you're sitting or standing. It is this reason that the traditional gurus would meditate sitting in lotus fashion on the ground. When both energies are present and moving, we call that Shivashakti current.

The rest of the chakras orient horizontally, like holes in a flute; as you change the flow of the air going thru a flute, you change the tone. As you change the energy moving through your chakras, you change the energy you put out. When Shivashakti energy is balanced and flowing through your chakras, it's like blowing the flute especially hard. There will be no other option but for the flute to change the sound of the world around it. Stretching the analogy back to chakras, when the Shivashakti current is moving powerfully through your body, you are changing the very energy of the air around you. At the very least, you are changing your perspective on the world.

Whether that change is pleasant or unpleasant depends on a lot of variables; namely what TYPE of energy being put out, which greatly depends on the environment around you. In a downward spiral, it can become a vicious cycle. A bad environment creates a negative mood, a negative mood provokes negative energy broadcasting, which affects everyone around you, then interacts with you and put you in a worse mood.

However, Tantrics take control of our own energy flow, and thereby control to a large extent, our reactions to the world around us, and by extension, how others perceive both the situation and us.

When we pay attention to the here and now, we have more energy available at any given moment. The sensory world is full of light waves, sound waves, and textures that are energy sources for our bodies. We evolved to be a part of this universe of light, sound, and texture. Paying attention to the Here and the Now adds energy to your system and helps raise your vibration. If you do it with no emotional connection, no decisive feeling, you will find that the energy boost is as clean and powerful as that of Pranayama breathing. Assigning any sort of value to what you are seeing merely distracts you and reduces the amount of energy you are getting out of the moment. Simply pay attention to everything like you did in the Fruit and Flowers exercise.

Your physical energy increases when you are here and now because you are actually paying attention to the Matter and Energy within your own environment. Everywhere Shiva and Shakti meet, energy increases. Absorb it. Use it. Broadcast it back into its environment with a more positive spin on it. You know how it works now.

Pure Shivashakti energy causes no harm; it only corrects things that are not on the right path. However, if you have messed up chakras, you are going to be broadcasting messed up energy. Your goal, then, is to run Shivashakti energy as cleanly as possible, without the sticky fear-blocked chakra residue.

"Ok, Sienna," you ask, "What does this have to do with the Kundalini?"

Why we do Karezza:

Doing Karezza shows you exactly how much energy can be stored in the chakras. This is necessary for your progress toward Kundalini awakening. When you finally get through the next few exercises, and get Kundalini up and running, your Karezza training will help you handle it safely.

During the Kundalini meditation, you gather up energy in the bottom chakra, and bring it intentionally toward the crown, essentially bringing Shakti energy UPWARD, making it meet the Shiva energy coming down from the crown. It is this upward moving Shakti energy that we call Kundalini. The goal is to bring that Kundalini energy all the way through your body to the crown, to balance out the Shiva energy you've always been pulling down. That gives both Shiva and Shakti energies to all 7 chakras. Without prior Karezza practice, this can overload your system very easily.

The mythology states "The Kundalini Serpent is a cobra snake wrapped around the base of the spine 3 times." There is no scientific support for this statement. However, many of the books written in 'twilight language' mention "serpents," "cobras," and "snakes." (Egyptian Pharaohs wore headdresses with snakes, supposedly adopting a similar mythology for a similar reason.) Aside from its obvious association with the human penis, the cobra snake symbolizes the Kundalini at peak; you will feel your energy expand around the top three chakras, somewhat like the hood of a striking cobra, when Kundalini is at its highest vibration.

The idea that it is 'wrapped 3 times' could refer to the difficulty in bringing the energy all the way to the crown; it takes most people at least three tries. The ancient texts are also very clear about Kundalini being feminine energy. It is entirely referred to as "she."

If you've had success with the Abyss ritual, your psyche is prepared for Kundalini; it is no longer necessary to push yourself with Karezza as your engine. We will be returning to Karezza, with a twist, later on. If, however, you are still struggling to make it to 28 minutes of Karezza meditation, or you are not prepared to approach your Abyss, you should continue with those exercises until you have reached that goal.

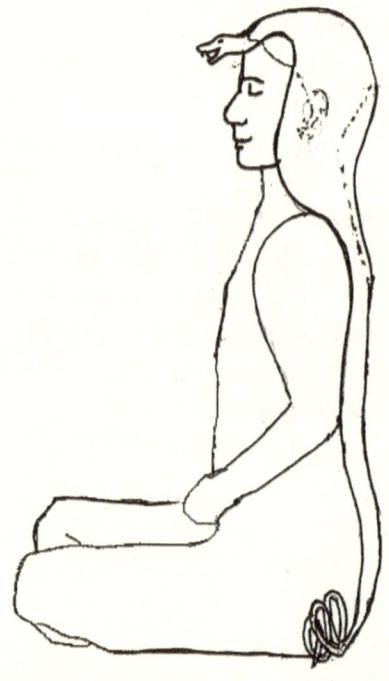

The Kundalini Serpent is the path up the spine
and out the third eye.

The Kundalini path

The Kundalini Path (synonymous with your Chakra Path, Shivashakti path, or Shushumna) is not your full body, but merely your spinal cord. Yes, that tiny little strand of nerve cells running inside your vertebra is the center of your energetic being. Its connection to "survival of the self" is apparent, as it's the first thing to develop in our embryonic state. The spine, like the rest of the nervous system, operates on pure ionic energy. Minute molecules flipping their electrical charge from slightly negative to overwhelmingly positive in a fraction of a millisecond produces the impulses that travel up our spine. This flip is highly contagious, and during Kundalini arousal, it sets off a rapid chain reaction of molecule flipping that becomes the Kundalini current.

It is quite possible to flip those molecules too far into the positive, and cause a runaway reaction that creates havoc in the body, brain, and aura. This is what we call ' Kundalini overload', and no matter who you ask, it sucks. The Karezza exercise sets up our nervous system to receive Kundalini without over stimulation.

What does Kundalini overload look like? It's emotional outburst without control or reason. Kundalini overload can cause a lot of tension and anxiety issues. However it can also make ordinary problems seem overwhelming, which then causes us to broadcast negative energy, which in turn creates a horrible reaction in the universe around us. So, this is a condition to avoid if possible.

If there are things that are going on that are crisis oriented in your personal life, do NOT attempt the Kundalini meditation. Wait until all crises have been averted. If, however, most things in your life are relatively predictable, it's time to work on this. The meditation for Kundalini follows in italics. Feel free to copy it and carry it around with you for meditation. Keep working on your chakras until you are familiar enough with them to understand what it feels like if one isn't functioning correctly. This will also help you avoid Kundalini overload.

When Kundalini is successful, you will find a lot of changes in your world. First, your workload increases on all fronts. Keep in mind that it will *never* increase to the point that you cannot handle it. (WRITE THAT DOWN SOMEWHERE!) You may find you have to prioritize your time, though, because you still only get 24 hours per day. The level of work you find yourself putting out, whether it's for money or pleasure, will definitely increase until you are at your full capacity of getting stuff done. Be wary of new projects while working on Kundalini.

Also, your instinct/intuition/psychic ability will increase. You will find that this skill has made enormous leaps once you have succeeded at Kundalini. This is because Kundalini does only one thing for your body, but that one thing is everything. It gets all of your neurons from the brainstem on down to fire all at once. And a good portion of the brain will go off as well. (This is exactly what psychologists hope to achieve when they apply electro-convulsive shock therapy, except this is much more natural and kind to your system!) As you might guess, all this natural neurological firing takes time, which is why we experience Kundalini in waves, rather than one big explosion.

These experiences of 'waves' really are ups and downs of your ions flipping, recovering from the flip, and then flipping again. Because of this, you get a wave of ionic electricity within the physical body like an ocean wave. The sheer force of these waves propels the energy outward from the body. Machines like EEG's can sense this wave, and you may find yourself screwing up streetlights and radios now and then. Most people ignore it, but humans and animals can usually detect it some way, even if subliminally. Yes, kittens will love you.

This is why we do Kundalini meditations in the privacy of a consecrated and separated space--so that we don't screw up anyone else's energy. How does that lead to extra work and precognition?

The extra work thingy is easy: you are attracting it to you with the extra energy you are putting out. You're broadcasting, "I can do anything." Therefore, the Universe gives you anything it can for you to do. Especially things that make life worthwhile…like art, loving children and animals, good food, sex, and the like.

What about precognition? That takes more explaining, but keep in mind that Kundalini energy creates a wave from your body outward.

Time & Tantra

Time IS nonlinear. I would say that Tantrics have known this for centuries, except that they "know" this for centuries. Most people see

Time as littered by solid things that once existed, still exist, or will exist in the future. These things are physical, like tables and chairs, wars and famines, and people we used to know. However, Einstein proved that Time is a by-product of gravity, matter, and mass, not an original substance that the Universe had to deal with before its creation. So, what about the parts of the Universe where there is no matter, thus no mass, thus no gravity? Is there no Time as well?

You see that looking at Time as a linear subject becomes problematic in the face of Einstein's magick...er, uh, science. That leaves us with no perspective on time that really works for us. Time to step out of familiar perspectives of time!

Ancient peoples like the Mayans, Egyptians, Celts, and ancient Tantrics had individually different concepts of time, which apply very well to what we have learned so far.

Consider this: if there were no Time, then everything would exist all at once. And so it does, outside any respectable gravity well. Unfortunately, we're stuck in a gravity well that has broken things down so that only one thing can exist at any point in time/space at any given moment. If we could step out of the gravity well, then we could literally see everything existing all at once. However, to get to a place where there is no Time means to go somewhere that there is no matter, and physically nothing to see. There is physically nothing.

How do we get from the surface of Earth, where gravity sucks and time blows by, to a state where there is nothing but we can see everything all at once? Kundalini. In this state, at that moment of explosion, we are in a state of timelessness. We are no longer physical. The outward wave of Kundalini gains the Naked Flame all the momentum it needs to boost the internal "I" energy out of the physical body and out of the gravity well. Your Naked Flame winds up in a place where there is nothing. This place is where everything exists all at once. In that moment, the internal "I" energy downloads as much information as it can from the Universe, before dropping back into the physical body (still recovering from the Kundalini wave...). But, the information remains. Plus, the link to that headspace remains, too. You can train yourself to get back there just by going there once.

After you have activated Kundalini energy the first time, it changes your cells to accept more energy the next time. And more after that. Each time it gets more intense, you gain a higher carrying capacity for the energy, and a longer time in the state of timelessness. I haven't found the end of that cycle in 15 years of practice. Each time I sit down to do the Kundalini meditation it gets more intense. It's like learning to surf; you can tackle bigger and bigger waves as you gain skill with practice.

As you change your system with Kundalini, you'll find that accessing Time is not only effortless, but also difficult to avoid. The knowledge of which tree will eventually become a chair that will eventually burn in a fire pit becomes more than easy; it is information you simply have in your mind. It's as easy as knowing your own name. You KNOW that the tree/chair/ash exists in one of those states at a given moment, and you know the sequence it should happen. All it takes is to know that it's a tree today, and you can be pretty damn sure it will be a chair next year and ashes 10 years after that, especially if you've already seen it in that state. The exact "dates" of happenings are still fuzzy with this perspective, but it's good enough for you to be able to forecast much of your own life.

The biggest problem is not turning yourself into a freak show with it. Careful choices of words are important here, and the True/ Kind/Necessary perspective is invaluable. Don't make statements that cause people to say, "How do you know that?" You're just going to "see" it.

What about the bad stuff?

Okay, so in seeing the future, you might see things you don't want to see, things you think you can prevent. You'll know which ones you can and cannot change simply by recognizing the outcomes as overly positive or overly negative for the whole community at large. Remember, here's no such thing as a free ride; knowing the bad is the price we pay for knowing the good. Don't screw your social life up by telling someone what you see in the Space Time Continuum. Listen and wait for the request for advice. Offer your knowledge as "you know, you might want to look at it this way." Cage your words carefully.

This comes across as increased "psychic awareness," but again, it's just the human being at its best. You might not know what those flashes of insight are about, and it's a very bad habit to make guesses based on this extremely limited information. Be quiet and watch, and you will find you can predict more than you thought possible. You might want to write them in a journal, just to prove to yourself that you're not nuts.

If you listen to your instinctual "hits," you will find that you can steer your life fairly painlessly if you just listen every day to that instinct. Eat only what your body wants. Sleep only when tired. Don't have sex just because the opportunity to screw presents itself. When your intuition says "turn right" don't ask why, just do it.

One major warning about opening up these psychic channels: It is possible for you to pick up uncomfortable energies from people around you. If you start feeling energy that is not yours, not true, or not pleasant, recognize this for someone else's energy you are attracting, and ground it out of your system.

Exercise: Kundalini raising

Set aside at least on hour alone without interruptions for this exercise. Create a sacred space and sit comfortably on the floor, arms and legs uncrossed. (Remember to keep your arms and legs uncrossed throughout the duration of the exercise.) Use the "Ham Sah" mantra that you learned in Pranayama. Do not speak it – just hear it in the breath. Make sure you are relaxed and not forcing your breath.

When you are comfortable with this, visualize the air in the room as breathable light. With each "Ham," you should imagine the light entering up through your nose, past your third eye, around the inside of your skull, and down your spine to the lowest tip of your coccyx (tail) bone. You should not feel the energy "hop" or avoid chakra points. Hold your breath as long as comfortable then exhale "Sah."

As you exhale, you should visualize light of a slightly different shade going back up your spine, pushing out the light you inhaled. This second light is the very beginning of your personal Kundalini energy. The light should follow the same path, up your spine, over the top of you head, and out your nose. As it goes, you should hear the "Sah" part of your breath stretched out for a few long seconds. Continue this for about 20 minutes; Haaahhhhmmm- hold – Saaaaaahhhhhh – rest – Haaaaaaaahhhhhhhmmmm – hold. You may find your base chakra becoming warm, and notice yourself physically relaxing at the end of the 20 minutes, if you are doing it right.

Once you have this part down, and can do it comfortably, don't hold your breath at the base of the spine, but just pause a moment. Then, using your stomach muscles, you should release the breath in short bursts, hearing "sah, sah, sah, sah, sah," as many times as it takes before your lungs empty. Keep up the light visualizations; the light will jump with the breathing. Repeat this for another 20 minutes. Haaaaaaaahhhhmmm, sah sah sah sah sah. You will be able to see or feel your Kundalini energy increase with each breath.

If you begin shaking and jerking, know that this is a normal reaction to the increased energy in your system, and you should not fight it. (Like a shiver down the spine, it is called 'kriya' and is totally involuntary and natural.) Don't scare yourself into stopping the exercise at this point. Soon the jerking motions will stop and you may begin moving in a very fluid fashion, somewhat like a serpent. You will not be able to hold still after this point, and you shouldn't try.

The energy will increase to the point where a large force builds up to your third eye chakra. Once you have this flow at what feels like maximum capacity, CONTINUE FOR AS LONG AS YOU CAN. When you finally release the energy, BE SURE YOU CONCENTRATE ON PURE LOVE. If you have no blocks, you will get the experience of a lifetime from this exercise. Do not be shocked at anything your physical body does or where your mind goes when you release the energy. If your mind wants to wander at this point, allow it. It will open you up to pheeling energy as you never have before. Remember to ground out any residual energy before coming out of the sacred space.

If you have stuck chakras, or knots, you will give up after a time, having only raised the energy to whatever chakra the knot lays in. It is vital for humans to have free-flowing energy to stay healthy in body and mind. Any knots must be untied. When you feel the knot or stuck chakra, STOP the exercise, let the energy subside, and ground the rest. Then remember which chakra the energy stopped at. It is in this chakra that the energy is blocked. I advise anyone who comes to this point to seek the advice of a Priest or Priestess of magick, or a counselor or guru of some sort.

Spontaneous arousal

It is possible for Kundalini to become aroused spontaneously due to external factors, such as emergencies, psychedelic drugs, extreme sports, and sexual ecstasy. Kundalini activates adrenaline in our system in times of trauma. We've all heard stories about people who can lift cars or move heavy things to save the life of a trapped person; these are not myths, they are the result of extra energy in the person's system, the natural state of Kundalini activation. We can assume for the most part that these people had no training in Kundalini yoga, and were simply following the dictates of spontaneous, instinctual, Kundalini arousal. Since Kundalini is a natural phenomenon, you can see how it evolved to help people survive in times of crisis.

> Kriya:
> Involuntary shivers and shakes in the nervous system that represent energy leaving the body.

During Kundalini arousal, the human body charges up its own battery and the energy takes the path of least resistance. Under ordinary circumstances, there is enough resistance in our chakras to keep our Kundalini energy at a relatively low (normal) level. When we are in a position to forget the ego all together, such as at the scene of an accident, or in the middle of orgasm, the chakras temporarily open up wide, and Kundalini may rise without our control, which is what most people fear about Kundalini. Humans don't like to lose control.

Kundalini is a potent tool, yes, but so are teeth. And like teeth, we must learn to use our energies correctly or they will not do their job. Warning people not to use their

> Spontaneous arousal:
> When energy levels raise in the body due to unforeseen situations or unintentional practice.

teeth is silly, and so it is for Kundalini as well.

Abyss or Kundalini First?

The Kundalini meditation and the Abyss ritual are truly complementary. Kundalini and the Abyss Meditation will help you step through the energy blocks of your chakras by working in tandem like a seesaw.

When you raise Kundalini energy, and bring the Serpent energy up to whatever chakra is blocked, it will stop. At that point, you can use the Abyss ritual to get that chakra unblocked. After that, you can try Kundalini again, and raise that energy up to the next higher chakra that is blocked. The Kundalini will help to show you where you need to work, and the Abyss meditation will help you get the work done. Remember, in the beginning of the book I said it might take 3 years to get through all this. You'll spend most of that time clearing the chakras.

Warning: Excessive Kundalini in one chakra will create it's own cure!

If you push too much Kundalini energy into a blocked chakra, the situation needed to unblock your chakra will occur on the physical plane. In other words, you will activate the lessons that you need. For example, if you have a communications block, and you pile up Kundalini energy behind your throat chakra and you will radiate "communicate with me!" Opportunities to speak out will show up all around you. If you ignore those, then you may find a crisis ensues in which you will be forced to speak out or suffer something unpleasant. If you ignore that, the crisis will occur and you'll find yourself doing nothing but complaining about repetitive crises in your life. This is not communicating; in street vernacular, they call it "bitching" and nobody likes to hear it. The solution is to find the block in your communication system and change the energy you are radiating before it creates any negativity on the physical plane.

If your base chakra is blocked, you must deal with that first before any others, or Kundalini will go nowhere. This means you will have to tackle any sexual and survival issues first. If you take the example above, and apply it to that base chakra, you can see that opportunities will change; you will find more opportunities for real connections, and act on them (or screw them up) accordingly. Remember to relax and be here now when doing any work on any chakra--this gives you the ability to break up any blocks, as well as the knowledge of any underlying issues.

Putting a little extra energy into a known block can help shine a light on the causes of the block, especially if you know there will soon be situations that will force you to confront your blocks. For example, working through a sexual block may open up opportunity for group sex, or give you alone time with a particular person so that you can open up to them, or mess with your birth control method. Figuring that out before it becomes a crisis stops the crisis from occurring (things like STD's, arguments, or unintended pregnancies), or lets you know that a pleasant situation is at hand, so that you can relax and enjoy it to its fullest potential.

It is up to you whether you use Kundalini to open up the channel to the Abyss, or if you use the Abyss to clear the way for Kundalini. My suggestion is to use them in tandem, gently approaching one then the other, until you work through all of your chakras. If you know the results of both, you will be able to work through them safely and sanely.

Eventually, your chakras should be so clear as to be able to bring up the Kundalini energy in three simple breaths. Why? Because, this skill gives you control over your body, mind, and energy that is necessary if you are going to carry the higher vibrations of the advanced rituals of Tantra.

So Many Men, So little Time:

A student relates:

"My first attempt at Kundalini occurred while I was between relationships. I had gone to the Midwest to visit my mom while grieving a messy divorce to a short-lived marriage. While there, I found myself resisting the advances of three other men. I wasn't interested in sex, nor was I interested in doing anything but getting my own head together. When my teacher suggested that I work on my sexual balance, I resisted that, too. Who cared about sex when my world wasn't going to straighten out until I straightened out? I needed a job, a plan, and a future without relying on men, and I knew that sex with any man would create even more problems for me. Still Sienna insisted that I try the meditation.

I felt as if I could not raise the energy beyond my own navel, which discouraged me from trying it a second time. However, within three days of trying that first meditation, all three of my potential suitors contacted me to say that they understood my predicament and would all be patient with me. One even drove 50 miles one-way to tell me this in person!

Less than a week later, I got news that I would have to return to the West Coast very soon. I decided to meet with each guy in person to let him each know that the game was over. All three of them requested--and received--the classic "goodbye fuck." Much to my surprise, I enjoyed every one of them more than I thought I would.

As soon as I hit the West Coast, I did the meditation again. This time the energy came all the way to my heart. The very next day I dropped in on a long-time male friend who was very glad to see me again. We started dating, and eventually I had a long-term stable relationship with him.

Train your brain

For every mindset that we wish to be able to bring back to us, all we need to do is install a "trigger." This comes in handy to recall the Kundalini energy. Once you have brought the Kundalini energy up to your crown chakra, all you need to do is be intently focused on a visual, audio, or textured item to set up a trigger. Then, in the future, the same color or pattern will help you recall the Kundalini mindset achieved. Smells work even better for this purpose, which is why all Temples have incense.

This programming process is so immediate that it's difficult to grasp that it's not about learning anything. It's about putting the basic components of our nervous system to the use in a natural fashion. Learning comes in many different forms.

You can easily recognize your triggers, once you are aware of the concept. Like candle light dinners invoke romance, the triggers we set up when we meditate will stay with us for a long time if we practice with them regularly.

Side Effects of Tantra:

The physical side effects of Tantra include increased appetite, reduced need for sleep, craving for healthier foods, and a general feeling of having more energy. One should expect this sort of change when starting any new discipline that increases your oxygen intake, such as new exercise plans or quitting smoking.

However, it takes a little more effort to get comfortable with the mental side effects of practicing Tantra. It is common to find you suddenly have the ability to project energy beyond your aura, such as tapping someone on the shoulder even though the shoulder is beyond your reach. Or speaking the same words at the same time with someone else. Or making amazing catches, miraculous saves, or averting small disasters. These minor, seemingly "magickal" feats are nothing of the sort. They are the result of the human being at its fittest form, like pitching a no-hitter, running a 3 minute mile, or walking a tight-rope are nothing more than a very talented, very trained human working within the perimeters of natural human ability.

It's very normal to get visions and information you have no physical access to, hear other people's thoughts, pick up other people's feelings, see ghosts, feel spirits, get vibed out, freaked out, spooked out, moody, broody, and paranoid when you first get your energy open and Kundalini flowing. However, if you recognize that this is a side effect, and it's merely there to point out where your fears are, you will see that it can eventually be helpful.

Nothing that is not physical can hurt you. If you think about it, since the Naked Flame IS non physical, then NOTHING can really hurt the REAL you except for yourself. If you pay attention, there is nothing you can accidentally do that would create much harm. In other words, there is nothing to fear but fear itself.

To make these visions and oddities be more productive than scary, you must first notice what common themes are running through your experiences. There truly are common themes; but you must interpret them according to your knowledge of your own psychology, by using the flower bud meditation, the Abyss ritual, and any other diagnostic tools you have in your power. Once you discover where your fears lay, you can work on deprogramming them as well. No ghost, energy, psychic vampire, vibe, emotion, or non-physical being is going to derail you if you are acting with Truth, Kindness, and Necessity.

Exercise: No Fear: Meditation for Crappy Days

As you might have guessed by now, if Kundalini energy is awakened before the energy centers have been properly cleared and a student gets physically and psychically unbalanced, the negative traits become amplified (neurosis or other anxieties, etc.) and reflect back to the person's reality. This is unpleasant and unbalancing. What is a simple way to get rebalanced?

First, let me state clearly that I've never heard of anyone going so far off the deep end with Kundalini that they took their own life. These are myths perpetrated by those who did not have enough knowledge of what they were getting into. If one is aware of this energy, and one is playing with this energy, one is also aware that when something goes wrong you must DO SOMETHING ABOUT IT. They typically go back to their teacher, the book they read, or the source of the information that they received. Or they seek out new sources. If you have nobody to turn to immediately, try this:

When you notice something is going "wrong", stop and feel the energy of what's "wrong". Did you loose your job/honey/house? Did someone get angry with you for no reason? Did you wreck your favorite car/shirt/recording? What was it that hit you as negative? This is the feeling that you work with.

Take your most "wrong" feeling to it's most complete. Give your body, mind, and spirit permission to really feel the most negativity that can fit in your system. Tell yourself "This is the worst it can get." Really wallow in it, feel free to feel totally horrible about it, allow worst-case scenarios to trample thru your head. Say to yourself "This is part of the Human Experience, which I am here to participate in."

Realize your system will not let that energy go until it knows you have really experienced it. Cry, punch pillows, kick cans, whatever it takes to get that energy to move thru your system and OUT. Experience it to it's utmost. Avoid blaming others for what they did to contribute to the negativity, avoid looking for cause or blame. This is all about YOU really experiencing this stuff. That's all the cause you need.

Once your system has tired of this feeling, it will try to make you feel better by moving your thoughts to other subjects. Stop yourself form blaming someone or something else for the situation, and recognize this as the "done" point. When you find your thoughts naturally drifting toward the positive side of the situation, or trying to take an active approach to the problem itself, check with yourself to see if you are done with feeling like crap. Go ahead and ask yourself "Am I done feeling this bad yet?" If you are not, bring yourself back thru worst- case scenario visualizations, pulling the energy from the front of you and out your back until it's gone. Grief, loss, and pain are part of the Human Experience, and we all go through them eventually.

If you are done, and you cannot force any more negativity through your system, then do this:

Try Pranayama for a few minutes, allowing yourself to only focus on the Here and Now and recover from the previous negativity. When you catch your thoughts drifting, bring it back to your breathing. With each breath, allow the negative headspace to flow out with your exhale, and allow new insight and light to come in with your inhale. As you are sitting and breathing, realize that Here and Now you are fine. Here and Now, you are alive, heart beating. Whatever forces

*are playing upon your outer life are not going to be as effective if you
can be Here and Now at any time you want.*

*Because Here and Now only hurts when you're not paying
attention, or when you didn't learn what you needed to learn earlier.
When you find this sort of thing happening to you, your energy is not
balanced. Go back to the Karezza exercise and allow yourself a few
good orgasms to help clear the energy as well. The point is to get it
out of your system, and put your body back into balance.*

The use of Kundalini energy is two-fold. The first time you bring
up Kundalini to the fullest, you will have an experience of clear energy
flow. All times after that, the Kundalini acts as a maintenance tool,
allowing you to shake off minor negativity, pointing out where major
negativity is likely to hit next, and allowing you to take preventive
measures before dealing with the physical necessity of the energy
you are putting out.

There is nothing to fear in your own energy. There is nothing
you can bring in which you are not prepared to deal with. You can
only create the opportunity to hurt yourself to the extent of your
own ability. As you gain more power, you also gain the ability to do
damage to your own system. Hopefully, you also gain the wisdom to
know how to avoid it.

One more note about fear: If you look at your greatest fear, and
then look at your greatest desire, you will find that they connect to
the same chakra. If you ask yourself the "why" of this, and look for
common themes, you will find yet another key to unblocking your
chakras.

Why bad things happen to good people:

You will not suddenly find yourself at the center of a great tragedy
unless you draw it to yourself, OR if you are in the wrong community
that is drawing negativity to itself. The only scary things you will
draw to yourself as an individual are things that you must deal with
in this lifetime. This means you DO have the skills and tools to deal
with whatever comes your way.

Many people have a hard time grasping this concept due to "bad
things happening to good people." What they fail to understand is

that Karma works on all levels of social structure, as well as the individual. There is 'family', 'community', and 'national' Karmic patterns as well. While understanding that the people who die in wars, hurricanes and disasters are typically 'innocent' of any wrongdoing, their deaths always serve a purpose for the community around them to learn an awful lesson. The only thing more terrifying than death for most Americans is being responsible for other people's deaths. This is the basis of the "Blue Tantra" approach; Community means as much as partnerships to us.

There are people who are born into adversity, who have no choice but to struggle all their lifetimes. They, too, have a purpose, if only teach their community how to behave kindly.

Yes, all Karma causes pain if you do not learn from it quickly enough, and sometimes lessons come on large scales. Individuals sometimes do carve themselves very difficult paths in order to learn lessons, but also, sometimes people serve to be the lesson to others.

We all take turns having nasty things happen to us. Someone somewhere must suffer, or we would not be motivated as a society to make corrections. So, when you ask "Why do bad things happen to me?" the answer is very simple: it's your turn.

Groundwork

White: Kundalini meditation (earlier in this chapter).

Red: Full Experience during Sex: No, you cannot simply transfer the Karezza exercise from White to Red without further instructions, however, the next time you get sexual with your partner, slow down the action. Be fully in the here and now, and watch what your bodies are doing from the inside. If something feels good, enjoy it for how it feels rather than think, "it would feel much better if..." See if the change in focus changes the outcome of the sexual experience for you.

Blue: It is difficult, if not impossible, to raise Kundalini as a group. However, by now, if you have been doing these meditations as a group, you have figured out who has chakra blocks where, and which members are going to have harder times opening up. It is possible to work on these blocks as a group with the "no fear" meditation above or by traditional group therapy methods which are available just about anywhere. One need not have a professionally trained therapy mediator if working as a coven or an intentional family; one only needs to have someone to direct the flow of conversation. You can transfer that role between members or use a 'talking stick' format. The only rule is that everyone comes in with the same goals; to open up to each other verbally, with support, about our own past traumas and pains, and move on. However, as a community, you must be willing to open up to each other, in pain or in joy. This activity will create tighter bonds between group members than existed before.

Chapter 5:   Bhakti and Bhoga

Bhakti

Bhakti translates as "Devotion." Bhakti is the act of returning thanks, gratitude and sacrifice to a Deity of your choice. There is a saying in the some Tantric schools of Tibet: "Mantra, Yantra, Yoga, Bhoga, Bhakti, Shakti!" Which translates, roughly, into: Meditate on Colors, Sounds, Physical Feelings, Joyous activity, and Devotion to a Higher Purpose, and the Kundalini Serpent will rise! Bhakti in ancient Tibet included kneeling before an altar to one of the hundreds of pantheon Deities. For Americans, however, pantheon-type Deities are not truly our style and kneeling to anything is pretty much out.

This is where the American paradigm freaks out on Tantra. Many Americans, especially those raised in Abrahamic religions, fear that the act of Bhakti—kneeling before a pictured Deity you don't believe in—would either constitute a sin, or mere foolishness. Still other westerners balk at the concept of kneeling before a deity because of their scientific mindset and their absolute atheism. How can I be grateful to some other force for my great job and my great family if I did all this myself without any help?

Bhakti, for the purposes of your training, does not need to be an external thing. You can turn Bhakti around and give it back to yourself. When you are enjoying the fruits of your own labor, it is possible to be grateful, thankful and sacrificial to yourself, and to be your own personal Higher Power. The Heart-cave exercise was a good example of that.

If the concept of "worship" doesn't sound good to your American paradigm, think of the feeling you have for the smartest person you know. Or the respect you give the person who has the most social connections. It's the gratitude you have for a family member who is at your side when you are ill. All of these feelings rolled into one; that's Bhakti.

The spark of life within any human is a miracle worth worshipping. Your father left millions of sperm within striking distance of you're mother's egg; you came into existence as the one that won the race. Is that not a miracle enough?

Gender and Tantra:

Heterosexual, one-on-one partnership sex is the most common form of sex, but it is not the only form. The Naked Flame is non-gendered, and there truly is no duality in nature. There is no consistent either/or about the "XX" and "XY" 23rd chromosome—some people have XXY, XYY, XXX, or simply just an X. If the hormonal balance is upset during pregnancy, some people will be born with a male body and female characteristics and desires. Society labels these people "homosexual", but they are human, and they also have the Naked Flame within them. Is that Naked Flame for them Male or Female? It's the same as it is within you: genderless.

One of the hallmarks of being ready for Red Tantra is that the student is able to work with both the Shiva and Shakti side of his/her personality. This requires that you be comfortable with the attributes of all genders. There are times when females have to be tough; there are times when males have to be gentle.

Gender is the social outcome of a biological fact. There truly are more than two genders: Maleness and Femaleness fall across a spectrum, due to physical biological reasons, from the ultra-feminine female and the ultra-masculine male. When you consider the thousands of tiny changes necessary for an embryo to come out male or female in entirety, it's a miracle that there are not more people born outside of society's concept of "Man" and "Woman." As it is, approximately 10% of the population does not adhere to either of those categories entirely, be it in physical appearance, behavior, or personality. (see Westheimer).

Therefore, consider that you, as a distinct entity, need not conform to either gender in entirety. You may fall on one end of the spectrum comfortably, or you may enjoy living somewhere in the center. However, to activate your fullest capacity, you must be comfortable in any position on the spectrum.

Using the following exercises, get to know how it feels to be on the far end of the spectrum from your current position. You may learn things about yourself that have kept you from connecting deeply with others. You may find that you play hard to get, that you freeze up when aroused, or that you don't allow your lover enough time for his or her own needs. Accept this information as a necessary lesson, and take the necessary steps to clear your habits of these issues.

Pay attention to how you interact with people of other genders, and people of your own gender. Gender plays a huge part in the construction of your own ego; examine that carefully. It is only by chance and biology that you landed in the body you have, being the gender that you are. This is not the true "you." This is not the Naked Flame.

Exercise: Making Love to Yourself:

This is actually a two-part exercise. The first is to play-act with yourself as a different gender and pay attention to both sides of the gender coin. With everything you do, from getting up from a chair, to making phone calls, even eating, do it as if you were of the most opposite gender from yourself on the continuum. If you're a female, approach the day as a mal and vice versa. Try this for a few days, and see what epiphanies it brings on.

The other exercise requires you to approach the inner self as your favorite gender and make love to yourself. Go the whole way, from flirting to dinner all the way to completion of orgasm with masturbation. Realize what it is like to be your own lover. What have your past lovers had to contend with, when dealing with you? You are the Deity you've been waiting for.

See your Naked Flame in your mind's eye as the Deity that you are. Recognize how special and significant you are in your own existence, and worship yourself for that reason. Thank your intellect, your body, your mind, and your luck for putting you where you are today. Give yourself a gift. Worship yourself, inside and out.

Exercise: Chakra Egg Meditation:

Besides being the introduction to the art of internal Bhakti, the Heart Cave exercise in Chapter 2 will become another diagnostic tool for you to use when working through your Abyss issues. The Heart Cave meditation can actually be adapted to all seven chakras, simply by visualizing each chakra as an egg. Each egg contains yet another internal double, who differs from the physical you only slightly (depending on the subconscious message being embodied), and only in the context of the chakra where it lives. Each egg should be a comfortable, clean environment for each Inner Self you meet there. Each egg should be suitable for Bhakti worship of your self.

Meditation:

Take the time to check in with each chakra by visualizing it as an egg. Knock on the shell of the egg to see which part of you comes out or lets you in. Look at the condition of the space; is it organized and neat, or messy and unkempt? The conversations you have with the inner double of each egg will be positively revealing.

A Party in the Heart

"L" was a newly married woman who was taking my class along side her husband because they were not feeling as if their sex lives were fulfilling enough. L could not remember the last time she had an orgasm, and her husband had given up trying to satisfy her. It was with this mindset that they approached these exercises.

When L tried the Chakra Egg meditation, she found that all of the chakras were welcoming to her conscious attempts at getting to know them, except for the base chakra. For some reason, it would simply not let her in. Although she succeeded in the 28-minute touch exercise, she also reported that she had no problem giving up the 'pocket fantasy', as she had none.

Of her own accord, she returned to the Heart Cave, and one-by-one invited all the other Inner Selves into the Heart at once. The throat, third eye, fight-or-flight…all of the Inner Selves that she had already gotten to know were drawn into the heart cave in her meditation.

All of the inner selves showed up except for the base chakra self. To entice the base chakra into the group, she began playing music—sexy, wiggle-your-hips dancing music—and decorated the Heart Cave as if for a party. She then began dancing with all the other Inner Selves until her Sexual Self showed up at the entrance to the cave. L knew herself well enough to know that her Sexual Self was quite comfortable on the dance floor of a party or a club, 'shakin' it.' Soon, all seven chakras and her Conscious Self were dancing in the Heart Cave together. On the physical, in her meditative state, she found herself masturbating Karezza-style without realizing it. As the energy increased, she became more familiar with her Sexual Self, until she was able to achieve an intense orgasm.

While still focusing on the "party in her heart," L was then able to communicate with the Sexual Self in this environment. The response she received made sense in light of her marriage problems. Her Sexual Self was just waiting for something interesting enough to be active about. Her husband's attempts at sex, it seemed, were simply not exciting enough anymore to be enticing to her. Her Sexual Self gave L plenty of ideas that she and her husband were able to incorporate as new aspects of sexuality in their relationship. This Tantrically gleaned information probably saved their marriage in the end.

American Men:

There's a phrase coined by director Jackson Katz that defines how American culture socializes males in their childhood to hide their feelings—he calls it the Tough Guise. Katz shows in his videos how masculinity in America is "amping up" violence and power-over mentality while discarding the human feelings all men have.

The tough guise has an impact on Tantra in that it creates a shield that women cannot get through energetically, emotionally, mentally, or physically. To perform Red Tantra, one must connect with each aspect of one's partner. If women can't get through to men, then the energy does not connect.

American men are products of their society, subjected to negative actions if they attempt to step out of the roles produced for them. To speak truth, to be kind, to act only when necessary are the hallmarks of a Tantric Priest, and those concepts do not go well with the 'tough guise.' You cannot make love and war simultaneously.

American men practicing Tantra must recognize when that 'tough guise' comes out, and learn to remove it from their relationships with women, or Red Tantra will not work.

American Women:

Women have helped to perpetuate the 'tough guise' by allowing it to become so powerful simply by being silent bystanders for too long. American women learn from an early age to fear men, to jump when any man gets violent, and to prepare for anger if we argue or talk back. No one man need do this training; society does it.

This sort of programming also creates fears, which creates shields that are difficult to negotiate for Tantric rituals. Fear of violent sexual attacks, fear of being taken advantage of, fear of not being attractive enough, and fear of incompetence are programmed fears from the rest of society. Rape just one woman and two hundred women will change their routine. One unseen man can force an entire city block to go on lockdown. What a power trip!

Recognize that some fears you will encounter are society's programs. Male vs. Female violence is not an American phenomenon. To be sure, there are many countries where the gender balance is more unequal than here! However, to create a Tantric link between genders, we must truly understand all genders and all the fears, shields, and barriers each gender has regarding opening up to the love of others.

What's so important about Balance?

Many paths in magick include ideas of duality in balance. God/ Goddess, Yin/Yang, Light/Dark, Matter/Energy; even the Tree of Life in Kabalah is balanced. So, what's the big deal about Balance?

Humans think differently with the right side of their brains than with the left. According to modern neuroscience, the left side of your brain does reasoning and rational thought processes like math. The right side is more responsible for artistic thoughts, original ideas, and recognizing shapes. You can't balance your checkbook or dig a hole while thinking with your creative side, and you can't write a heartfelt letter or decorate your home while thinking with your rational side. Okay, you can, but they don't come out right. You will be dissatisfied with the results. Therefore, it benefits all Tantrics and energy-workers-in-training to learn to use both sides of the brain equally. By knowing which hemisphere is dominant, we can determine the style of learning that will be most effective for us, and we get another clue to deprogramming our mental habits.

There is also a dichotomy between conscious mind and subconscious mind. The conscious mind works on the social side of us that keeps us from blurting out "let's fuck" at the wrong moment. The subconscious or inner part of our brains is the part that houses our True Will, what we really should be doing. If they don't line up together and work in unison, you get very dissatisfied with your environment. Therefore, balance between conscious and subconscious brings one to the point of being able to enjoy our environment. (as in the tact to say politely, "I'd like to get to know you better" when "let's fuck" is on your mind.)

When someone uses all of his or her energy to bring about changes in consciousness, the human must be in balance between right/left and conscious/subconscious. If the consciousness is overriding any desires of the subconscious, those underlying desires will manifest in the outcome of the behavior. If the work requires the use of right brain thinking and you are stuck in a left-brain mindset, you will be dissatisfied with the results. How do you stay in balance through your daily life so you can be your best at all times? Here's a trick:

Stand up right now, wherever you are, and lift one foot. Make sure you are balanced then pay attention to the foot that is still on the floor. What is it doing? It's making tiny adjustments to keep your center of gravity where it should be. This is how we learn where our balance is. We make tiny adjustments to our paradigm as we live day to day.

We get out of balance when we make "always" or "never" statements, which stop us from adjusting to changing circumstances. If you ALWAYS need to have things a certain way, or if you NEVER react to a situation that requires reaction, will the Naked Flame be free? Examine your own behavior for Always and Never statements, and realize that there are times when those actions will not suit your needs. These absolute statements will keep your paradigm inflexible, unable to make those tiny adjustments necessary to keep yourself in balance. You may even find that when you challenge your Always and Never statements, you go way off balance! This is a big clue to examine your behavior.

We also can get out of balance when we try to push ourselves to do more than what we can do, or less than what we should do. Your physical balance will show you if your mind is out of balance; you can always test yourself by finding a curb to walk along, the top of a rounded rock to stand on, or simply standing on one foot. To be in balance within yourself is to be in line with your Naked Flame, allowing nothing to throw you off of it. To be in line with your Naked Flame is to be in balance with the Universe. You have the power to make your personal universe an easier place to live in, if you simply strive for balance, making those tiny adjustments to your paradigm every day, and give up on absolute statements.

Orgies! Orgies everywhere!

Say "Tantra" in America, and someone will think "Orgies!" The word brings to mind sexy, sexual, enticing, lewd behavior, and big piles of hot steamy bodies screwing with wild abandon. I would be lying if I said that these ideas were pure myth. They're not; indeed, Tantrics do have ritual orgies.

The point of these orgiastic rituals was to forget the earthly body and all the ego trappings that come with it. Ancient Tantrics would eat, drink, partake of mind-altering substances, and have sex with strangers, all to help remove the ego.

When you give your ego a temporary vacation, it needs to be in a setting where all other people are doing the same thing, or you become a problem to your community. This sort of "ego removal" in large groups would definitely lead to an outpouring of sexual energy, creating an orgy. The attendees of these rites understood their purpose, and only participated after they had intensely trained and practiced for years.

Tantra is a path which one must start at the beginning and work up from there. Just as a marathon runner didn't start training by running 100 miles, a Tantric can't start training in orgies.

What happens to a lot of 'self-taught' Tantrics is that they get stuck working the energy of one chakra, and they get a great rush out of it. If it's in a lower chakra, such as our sexual centers, the practitioners get an orgasmic rush that they've never had before because that sexual center has never opened before. What doesn't occur to most of them is that there are more chakras to clear.

Exchanging energy when the only open chakra you have is the lower ones (where most people start their training) leads one to a life of hedonism, wretched excess, and wallowing in lower, material-bound energies. It really feels good to have energy flood in and out of it after years of blockage, which is what happens in any serious sexual encounter, but that's only a distraction.

Afterward, when the beginner absorbs all the energy in his/her partner's base chakras, the student will feel powerful. This affect could last for days. It's really addicting, causing the practitioner to suck up more and more energy, even though the energy may not be clean. Some claim to be teachers so that others come to them and give up their energy willingly. Soon, instead of a holy order, they have a fan club.

What usually happens is that these people eat the Karmic return for their actions. They contract STDs. They find themselves rejected by their followers or psychologically unhealthy. Sometimes they fall into old patterns again, giving up the Enlightenment trail all together.

Sacred orgies did not include the type of beginner that only had one or two chakras open. They were for the more advanced practitioners who had been working on it for years, with all seven chakras open and functioning well. If you can imagine the orgies as being about communications, feeding, security, sharing meditations, and all the other chakra fields, you get a better idea of why Tantrics had orgies.

Unveiling what we are otherwise afraid to express, wallowing in pure joy and pleasure, relaxing, breathing it in, sharing it with a partner are all necessary steps in learning Tantra. To accept what our physical body is doing and to have our mind in control of it at all times is the goal of Tantra. Hedonism has its place, but it's not the whole story. Understand why the Tantrics hosted orgies before you fantasize—or worry! —about participating in them.

Bhoga:

Bhoga translates as "joy." A Bhoga meditation has the purpose of pure joy. We seek out and participate in all things that create joy in our selves, from sniffing roses to eating chocolate to sex. In the Bhoga experience, one asks oneself "What do I want now?" for a determined period. Your groundwork in this chapter is to perform Bhoga, which is the "Joyous Activity" part of the program. Oh, yeah!

Bhoga is the practice that has always given Tantra a bad reputation. It is for the activity of Bhoga that the ancient Tantrics participated in 'orgies' and 'sexual indiscretions.' They would feast on meat and sweets, drink all types of beverages, especially alcoholic, and participate in group sex from dawn to dawn, for a full 24-hour period. They would ignore all marriage vows, and any other sexual taboo, such as anal sex, or sex with sisters and brothers, for just this one day. To Western eyes in the early years of exploration, this was an abomination. To Tantrics, this was an act of allowing the Naked Flame to experience the joy of having a mind, body, and energy.

To do the Bhoga exercise, you must put yourself in a situation, maybe at a party, maybe just a weekend off at home, and ask yourself "What do I want now?" Do whatever you want. Be your self, eat, sleep, have sex or masturbate, chat, climb, jump, play, create. Make sure it's fun; make sure it's what the Naked Flame wants.

Do whatever your Spirit tells you to do. BUT…(and you knew there was a catch, didn't you?) check in with all seven chakras before you do anything. Make sure that every part of your body is saying yes, and that no part is saying no. This takes time to sort out in your mind, so you may find yourself quite contemplative during this process. Make your decisions slowly. Remember that the physical circumstances you find yourself in will set your limits for you. You cannot fly if you cannot grow wings, so don't try to do something that you're not physically capable of doing.

Many students make plans in advance of the actual Bhoga exercise, and are greatly surprised when it turns out differently.

Some have decided that they will indulge in different chemicals, or perform certain sexual activities, which they think will be joyful for all seven chakras. Usually, however, they have not thought it through. For all energy exchange has a price to be paid, and Bhoga has its lessons to teach. It never quite turns out as you think it will.

You may think you want that chocolate, and perhaps part of you does. Another part of you is aware that you are not in need of it. If you only listen to the part that wants it, you will be consuming a substance your entire being does not agree with, which leads to unhealthy conflict within you. Bhoga listens to the part that says 'no' as well as the part saying 'yes.'

You can do Bhoga with a partner, but the most impact from this exercise comes when you practice Bhoga alone or with a crowd of others also practicing Bhoga.

Learning from Bhoga:

Several years after T had begun practicing Tantra, she decided that her biggest obstacle to learning was her relationship. She was married for over 10 years, and questioning the need for monogamy in her relationship. An opportunity arose to attend a festival without her husband, and we happened to be hosting a Tantric Puja at that event. She decided that a Bhoga would help her make up her mind about her relationship.

After the Puja, we always give the attendees an opportunity to stay or leave and T decided to stay. A polite, attractive man approached her, and she had to ask herself, "Does all of me want this?" Her Naked Flame answered, "YES!" That night, she broke her vow of monogamy for the first time in 10 years. T and this stranger had sex all night long in every position imaginable. When it was over, however, she realized that sex with this stranger was not nearly as satisfying as sex with her husband. This wonderful polite and caring man just did not have the connection with her that she was accustomed to at home.

Arriving home from the festival, T told her husband what had happened. At first, he was angry and they split up. T was confused. Why would the Naked Flame say, "yes" to something that would hurt her marriage? She and her husband had long discussions that lasted for days. He explained his fear of her finding someone better than he assumed himself to be. She convinced him that there was no one who COULD be a better sex partner for her. The result was a renewed energy toward their marriage, and T's husband starting on the path of Tantra. T remains with her husband in a devoted relationship that stands to this day.

Groundwork:

<u>*White and/or Red and/or Blue*</u>: Commit yourself to at least 24 hours of Bhoga experience. A whole weekend is even better. Eat, drink, get intoxicated on life, and let yourself be as sensual as possible. Pay attention to what is flashing through your mind, and allow yourself to let it all hang out. For groups, try a weekend campout. For couples, a private night at home will do. However, stop and listen to every one of your seven chakras before you go forward with any action.

Chapter 6:   K+K

Introduction to Maithuna

The highest Red Tantra ritual is called Maithuna. Maithuna is physical sex that includes the energetic and spiritual union between a Priest and a Priestess, done in Tantric methodology. Maithuna includes penetration, but it is not just having sex; it is a union of Shiva and Shakti on the physical plane, which broadcasts that sacred energy everywhere in your life.

Maithuna starts with connecting the energy of your Kundalini with that of your partner's Kundalini. Once this has happened, you add the physical component with penetrative sex-- lingam inside yoni. Then, you prolong

> **Maithuna:**
> The ceremony that involves worshipping the partner, invoking Shiva and Shakti, and having physical sexual coitus.

the union by controlling your orgasm via Karezza methods. All this connecting and controlling boosts your energy (and your partner's energy) to its maximum capacity. It's like nothing else you've ever experienced.

To be ready for Maithuna, you must be able to control your entire system. You can't slack off on this homework and expect to be able to achieve true Maithuna. There is a limit to the amount of energy that your body can handle, and Maithuna is gets you to that limit. Getting into partnered rites when you're not ready can be dangerous. You will create enough energy to manifest exactly what your aura is projecting. At the very least, you will orgasm within the first few minutes, and not achieve the desired effect of prolonged and increased energy.

How do you know when you've reached the ability for Maithuna? When you have been able--solo--to maintain maximum capacity power and hold onto that state of mind for at least 28 minutes.

What does Maximum Capacity Power mean? It's that state you achieve right before you go over the edge of the cliff and into orgasm. Maximum Capacity = can't take no more. However, going into orgasm is definitely NOT the point of Maithuna. Once the orgasm happens, all the fun is over—the energy dissipates, the lingam is no longer happy in the yoni, and you can no longer achieve that high vibration. Remember, the higher you can vibrate, the healthier you become. The healthier you become, the higher you can vibrate.

To achieve a state where you can safely engage in Maithuna with another trained partner, without dropping into immediate orgasm, you must have three things:

Total control over Body, (Kundalini, Karezza)

Total control of Mind, (Focus, balance)

Total control of Actions (total understanding of your ego, and your freedoms).

True, Kind, Necessary

Gossip, lies, exaggerations, and deceptions are all such a big part of American communications that we have come to expect it. Entire magazines are dedicated to gossip, we know that the media news is exaggerated, and an honest politician is hard to find. Having to discern truth in other people's statements wastes energy, something that Tantrics try not to do. How can an American Tantric be honest?

Start by changing the way you communicate. Set an example for others around you speaking only what you mean. Think about the words you use. All communications should be True, Kind, and Necessary. If you stop yourself before you speak and ask yourself these three questions, you can be relatively assuered that any misunderstanding is on the part of the listener.

1. Is what I'm saying absolutely true? Do I know it to be true? If it is my opinion, did I preface it as such? Do I need to use better wording?

2. Is what I'm about to say a kind thing? Is it something negative that I think my audience will find interesting? If so, why am I speaking it if it is simply spreading unkindness?

3. Is what I'm about to say necessary? Am I talking about a

subject my audience is interested in or needs to know? Or am I just wanting to hear the sound of my own voice break the silence?

If your words do not adhere to "True, Kind, Necessary," then ask yourself why you must speak them. Chances are, you'll catch yourself with negative energy you don't want anyway.

Your next task is to discern what is true communication coming at you, and what is bullshit put on by society. This is an eye opening exercise; or at least an ear opening one. By listening for what is True, Kind, and Necessary, you'll find that sarcasm is a way of life for some people; they can't communicate any other way. You'll notice how often slang gets over used. ('pickup that fuckin' shit', when taken literally, is quite gross....). You'll find out who is too timid to come right out and ask for what they want, and exactly how they go about getting their needs met.

When you discover people who do not say what they mean, take them literally. Behave in such a way that their underlying meaning is lost on you, and act accordingly. Ignore sarcasm. Eventually, they will decide they must deal with you in a less evasive fashion.

To keep to the True, Kind, Necessary communication method will solve at least 50% of all communication breakdowns. The other 50% is not under your control—it belongs to whoever you are communicating with.

Thought, Word, Deed

Energy is not just an external or an internal affair; it's everywhere in everything we do. We can ride the wave of the energy around us, or we can fight that energy and be on the defensive with it. We can use chaos to shatter and disperse it, or intention to channel it. We can use it to heal, use it to harm, or just use it to glean information. One thing a Tantric will *not* do is ignore it or forget about it. Paying attention to the energy around us is what Tantric training is for.

The energy that is inside of you is the same energy that comes out of you. If you try to change that energy as it comes out, it lands flat, something is obviously wrong with it. Think about how you can tell if some people are lying. Or how we feel when we pretend to like something. Faking it only works on those who are not aware.

One of the goals of the Tantric is to match Thought, Word, and

Deed. The thoughts you think should be the same as the words you speak, and those should be the same as the deeds you perform.

To match up Thought, Word, and Deed is a big job. Most of us will walk around without this integration all the time. We think about sex at work. We think about food when we're driving. We worry about home, health, and finance, but we talk about the weather, celebrities, the news. We make promises we hope we don't have to keep, and we perform actions we know that we shouldn't.

To be a trained Tantric is to stop that particular behavior, and to get a handle on it. To "integrate" your thoughts, words and deeds. The easiest way to get a handle on that one?

Be here now. Think about what is directly in front of you. Talk about what is directly in front of you. If there's not enough to think about there, then go inside and think about the energy within you. Don't go off into what-if tangents; that's a waste of your energy.

When you have control over your own words, your own mental processes, and your actions, then you are ready to raise your vibration up as high as it can get. We call this the state of "Sarvata" or "Integrity." "Integrity" indicates you have integrated pieces of the whole. You are One piece—and that piece is under control of the Naked Flame.

Exercise: K + K

If you think Karezza was fun before, you ain't seen nuthin' yet. This exercise combines Kundalini serpent energy with the self-stimulation techniques in Karezza. Woo Hoo!

Begin this exercise nude, in the place where you typically practice Karezza. Read through the Kundalini breathing meditation one more time, and get into the "Ham-Sah" breathing while sitting up, spine pointed toward the ceiling. Get the light flowing up and down your spine, using the long inhale and many-short-exhales pattern. Do not use Karezza just yet. You might want to photocopy the Kundalini ritual from chapter 4 or take the book into temple with you, turned to that page.

When you feel the Kundalini serpent energy begin heating up your base chakra, pull that energy up to the next chakra, then the next and then the next. Get the serpent as high up as you can, all the way to the crown, if possible. You will feel very high; your nervous system will be in an uproar, and --this is the important point-- you will not be able to sit still.

At the point where you hit a threshold within your body, you will begin to feel jumpy, twitchy, and wiggly. Think of that feeling as static electricity that must leave your limbs. When you first notice this beginning, this is the signal to SHIFT GEARS.

Continue the same "haaaam-sah-sah-sah-sah-sah" breathing pattern, but RELAX into your Karezza headspace. If you can remain sitting with your spine straight up, great, but if you must lie down to relax completely, make sure you do not sever the earth/sky connections at the Crown and Base chakras. The light path will bend if you imagine it shaped like a sideways S, turning above your head and below your butt.

As you continue to keep the Kundalini energy running through your spine, begin self-stimulation with Karezza. Relax and let all of the twitchy electrical energy run down your spine and out your limbs as you become like putty everywhere--except one hand and your genitals. The BIG difference at this point from your typical Karezza exercise is the breathing pattern and the sheer amount of energy inside your system. All else is the same, you just have a lot more energy to let flow through you.

I would say, "End this meditation as usual, with a release of orgasm." However, if you do it right, the orgasm you have will be anything but usual. Allow yourself to float on the astral and receive instruction from your subconscious before you come down and ground.

Details: Do not cross your legs when you are sitting up. Put them out in front of you, or sit on the edge of a chair or bed with your feet on the floor. The Kundalini electricity will circle back around your legs instead of going up your spine if you sit cross-legged. Do not be shocked or surprised by anything your body does. Observe and take note. Remember to ground the energy out into the earth when you are done. See the grounding exercise in chapter 4.

Do not fall into any type of fantasy. Wherever your focus is when this energy releases will be exactly what manifests in your life. THIS IS NO MYTH! I recommend a focus such as "perfecting this technique" or "being the best practitioner I can be" or "Allowing me to try this again." Turn it back on itself. This will make your learning easier. Even "Wheeee! This is fun!" is better than pulling out your pocket fantasy.

If you were handling Karezza energy beyond 28 minutes, or even to 56 minutes, do not be surprised if you cannot make that mark now. In fact, don't be surprised if you can't hold the Karezza energy for even 3 minutes the first time. If you slip up and dump a load of energy from this exercise into the wrong place (i.e. some unwanted fantasy) write it down immediately, so you can spot it when it manifests. It's possible to control the manifestation, but it's not possible to stop it all together. Tantric energy will manifest no matter what you do, and this will be the most Tantric energy you've ever had in your system until now. The only thing you can do as a cleanup is control how it manifests.

Here are the numbered steps:

1. *Do this nude, in private.*
2. *Raise Kundalini energy to the crown of your head*
3. *Use Karezza to bring yourself to orgasm while relaxed*
    Do not use fantasy!
4. *Release energy to some safe focus.*
5. *Repeat as necessary*

How can it possibly work?

If you have attempted the K+K exercise, you will know that it changes your headspace as much as the two individual exercises did by themselves. These exercises make permanent changes to the brain, which affects the Ego, and the K+K exercise makes the biggest change yet. Why would this be so? What is in a simple breathing pattern to make such a big impact on one's ego? Or, more importantly to modern psychology, HOW is this possible?

Let's look at this scientifically. First, we know that the brain's ionic energy is detectable outside the skull; we'll just call it "aura energy." Any EEG specialist will tell you it's real, it can be interpreted non-invasively, and it comes directly from the brain. So what the hell good would such a property be in Evolutionary Theory if it didn't broadcast or perceive something about our environment, such as emitting or receiving human emotional states within groups?

We use the aura for advertising how we feel, and figuring out if the big ape next door is a threat. (Facial expressions are only so useful in such situations, because we can't always see faces.) When we are young and learning our socialization skills, we have no ego, we have to build it. When we watch someone laugh at something, we challenge ourselves to find the humor that another person found; we want to laugh too. When babies see someone crying, they discover that only some reactions to emotional pain are acceptable behaviors. But, we can't just "monkey see monkey do" that sort of thing; if that were the case, emotions would be very flat. We pheel it (as opposed to skin-sensation "feeling" it), and watch the drama unfold around us, and say "aha!" Even a baby who can't talk will cringe when an angry person is present...and file that experience away in his amazing grab-everything baby mind. A traumatized baby learns to associate that pheeling with trauma, and builds a natural shield around its aura to stop the pheeling. That shield becomes a "trait" in the baby's future personality.

The aura helps us build the ego, and is there to help us hang it on the outside, which covers up the brilliance in the Naked Flame. It broadcasts what we want people to pickup, and shields what we want to hide. The more things we fear or regret, the more we have to hide, and the thicker the ego. The thicker the ego, the less spirit driven, and the more greedy-physical-earthbound a person is.

All the while, inside each of us, the Naked Flame is fighting to stay alive and healthy while the ego tries to beat it down. In some, it is healthy and attempting to do its job of helping us evolve. In most, it hides, so the ego stays in control.

Whatever we are broadcasting will draw more of the same to us. If fear is shielding your ego, you will find fears will be at every turn. This is why we see people in patterns of repeated lousy relationships, repeated accidents, and repeated depression. The key to their health is to find what the Naked Flame is trying to do, so that the ego can participate instead of getting in the way.

That's the path for ordinary people, not for Tantrics.

Ordinary people can live their lives happily just by getting over the biggest of their fears and letting the rest go by. Tantrics can have absolutely NO FEAR. None. Why? Because each one obscures the Naked flame a little bit, and that is a waste of our energy. Remember: the goal of a Tantric is to have access to all of his or her energy at all times.

How does the K + K meditation help? It kicks the Naked Flame loose from its boundaries, allowing it to view the ego as an empty cage. It sends you to an astral place that hands you your own shortcomings on a silver platter. It takes your mind directly to the point of the biggest, meanest, ugliest fear/resistance/fear/resistance that you have, and puts it directly in your crosshairs. If you find your inner double in all the debris, you may ask him direct questions and get the straight up answers you can't get from doing ordinary meditations (I mean straight up, NO RIDDLES!) This is why I recommend getting to know your Selves in the Chakra Egg meditation. Unless you are in constant contact with them all the time, you will not think to use them at moments of highest vibrational rates.

Basically, you can visualize the K+K rite as taking the Naked Flame, shaking the dirt off the outside of it, and boosting it up high above the earth so that it gets a satellite's view of your life, and the ability to do something about anything you'd like to change.

Remember, this rite will also manifest all of those fears UNLESS you change the energy you are putting out ASAP. K+K shows you where those areas are *before* you get stuck with the karma.

In other words, if you know that there are issues you haven't tackled, this is like dropping a big bomb on them. My co-teacher called it "Cosmic Draino." Unless you actively put your energy into mastering the K+K exercise, (i.e. 28 minutes with both aspects happening) you won't have any more power in your hands than you already have. My question to you is: Are you satisfied with what you have now, or are you willing to go for more?

Shortcuts:

Pranayama. Karezza. Chakras. Kundalini. Bhoga. Bhakti. With all this difficulty, it's possible that you will be thinking "wow, I need an edge here…a shortcut…a way to make it easier." Well you do. You already have it in your hand…so to speak….

The K+K ritual is your shortcut. Each time you go into that meditation, and you get into that headspace, and you release that incredible amount of energy, you have a magickal weapon of mass construction. USE IT! Tack on the concept of "mastering the skills of Tantra." Or "perfecting this exercise" or "becoming the best me I can be." You can harness that magickal energy created from your learning to boost your learning. Turn it back on itself each time you do it, and you'll get through the learning process in record time.

A Musician's Mistake:

"J" was a male student and a drummer in a garage band, who had a beautiful and talented female lead singer. Although he denied having feelings for her, he went out of his way to promote her career as a member of the band.

As he approached the K + K exercise, he was also attempting to set up and promote the largest show his band had ever played. He spent weeks selling tickets and posting flyers. When he sat down with the K + K exercise, his focus for the energy release was to have "a successful concert." His previous record for Karezza meditation was well over 60 minutes, and he entered the K + K exercise with confidence.

According to his own words, J reached orgasm the moment he shifted from Kundalini to Karezza, barely even touching his own lingam. Less than a day after this K + K attempt, he became horribly ill, and was eventually diagnosed with mononucleosis and ordered to bed rest for over a month. He missed the concert all together and eventually left the band.

Because of his hidden love for the lead singer, and his fear that she would discover his attachment, his energy broadcast the worst of his fears and, as a result, shattered the masks he wore. If he had admitted his affection for her, even to himself or to a friend, he may have saved himself the trouble of getting sick and wasting so much energy on a concert he never played. Once he recovered from

---

> the illness, he was able to confess his feelings to the singer, who was touched, but not interested. She let him down easily, though, which helped him have more confidence for future relationships, and cleared up some of his chakras.

Picture this:

You & your Tantric Priest(ess), nude, in Temple. You start with eye gazing, looking deep enough to touch each other's soul. You wrap your auras around each other and begin syncopated Pranayama breathing, exchanging the energy between the two of you. Using this rhythm, you both bring up Kundalini energy, and begin exchanging the Kundalini between your chakras. Then you slip lingam into yoni, with plenty of natural lubrication. You are now inside of each other, but not moving hardly at all. Only the muscles of her yoni and the muscles of his lingam are in action. You relax and breathe, falling into a tranced-out headspace. Your partner does the same. Now you have Kundalini fired up and you are sharing it, and it is getting faster and faster as it circulates between you. You do not orgasm because of your Karezza training, and the energy continues to build.

And then...You are no longer you, but now you are the God and/or the Goddess; fully manifested. The energy rushes between you faster than you ever thought possible.

> Om:
> The seed syllable of the universe. A sound to focus on in meditation.

You are no longer human. You become Matter and Energy, and you activate that creative spark of the Universe, the Big Bang, and/or the first Om. You are One. The energy builds for what seems like forever...and then you hit that 28 minute mark...and then the 56 minute mark...and then the 109 minute mark...

I cannot tell you where this leads, because it is unique to each couple. However, you can consider this scenario as "maximum capacity power in motion." This is the Maithuna rite, and it's the goal at the end of your training.

Groundwork:

White: 28 minute Kundalini + Karezza (described earlier)

<u>*Red*</u>*:* The couples K + K exercise. One of you at a time should be the meditator, and the other should be the helper. Make sure you each get a turn in each position. The meditator starts the Kundalini breathing, while the helper sexually stimulates the meditator. You can use hands, mouth, or whatever, BUT the meditator must stay still and limp, totally relaxed. This may take practice to make 28 minutes, but I have a feeling that it's homework you can live with.

<u>*Blue*</u>*:* True, Kind, and Necessary communications: Within your community, and within any other human interaction, keep in mind the concepts mentioned in the paragraph above. Explain this concept to as many of your contacts as necessary to help you on your path.

Chapter 7:   The Tantric Field

Healing with the Tantric Field

Since Tantra is the only spiritual practice built for two, there are nuances that never appear in any other spiritual practice. The vibration in a Tantric Maithuna ritual is the highest vibration achievable by the human body.

The field created by two Tantric bodies vibrates so intensely that

> **Tantric field:**
> The energy that surrounds a person or a couple when practicing Tantra.

everything in it must be healthy. If it is not healthy, and you bring it into the field, it changes and becomes healthy. Sometimes that's a shocking thing to do. However, I have never seen any living thing surrounded by a Tantric field that did not show signs of growth and healing within 24 hours. It's really some amazing stuff.

If you begin overriding a smaller energy system with a larger more powerful system, the energy changes the flavor of what's around it. If a living thing has an imbalanced energy, and you put it into a Tantric field, the energy puts itself back into balance. A larger energy force will always overpower the lesser energy. Batteries work on this same principle.

This is also why heavy-duty negative or unbalanced energy, can, if given the opposite ratio, pushed balanced things into an unbalanced state. It works both ways. Therefore, if we're generating positive energies, then everything we put into it, including ours selves, grows, changes and balances. That's why we learn to heal ourselves in our practices, so that we can generate positive energy and help heal other people.

Many physical ailments have a "psychological" component. The newest budding branch of medical research is 'biopsychology'--that which concerns the mind-body connection. The ancients knew about this, and attributed this phenomenon to an imbalance in the chakras. You now know how to clear your own chakras, and their connection to the nervous system and the brain. When you run balanced energy with another individual, you broadcast that clearer, higher energy, forcing their chakras to align as well. Granted, it may introduce them to the imbalances that they need to work on, which can uncomfortable, but the healing is still taking place.

Healers such as dentists, massage therapist, acupuncturists, and general MDs who have studied Tantra have been able to add more energy to their work and get better results. They are still doing the same technical work they were doing, but they now can add an overwhelming amount of energy to the work. That makes any hands-on healing better, any emotional counseling work out better... it enhances any healing. People who study Wicca, Druidry, Reiki, or ritual magick will have more energy to throw at it for their spiritual practices, too.

It's very useful and applicable anywhere because it's something that our bodies do naturally. It's not an alien skill. It helps with music, art, sports, just about any endeavor a person can undertake. The only thing that stops you from vibrating and being your healthiest at any given moment is your own internal programming.

And you know the programmer, up close and personal.

Exercise: Chakra Sealing

To seal a chakra means to align your chakra with that of your partner's, and "seal" them so that the energy is directly connected while working with a partner. It can be something as simple as a kiss or a touch, but you want to make sure that you acknowledge each chakra on your partner (and vice versa) before going into Red Tantric rituals. This keeps your chakras focused where they belong, instead of allowing the energy to dart left and right.

A touch is all you really need to remind the energy where to go. If you do the Puja ritual (in the next section of this chapter) before you begin, it will suffice for chakra sealing. You can mark them by writing symbols on the skin, or you can play with the elaborate old rituals in which all the energy centers are painted on the body. It's just opening up each chakra, making sure it connects to your partner's equivalent chakra in return.

The more you are connected to the partner you're working with, the easier the chakras will seal. If I am working with a student, there's always one chakra that doesn't want to connect at all, because we're not all that close. With my sexual partner, it's an automatic thing once we get turned-on to each other. It's hard to not connect with him.

Do one chakra at a time, both partners in turn, simply because it's easier to spot mistakes that way. The order you seal them in really doesn't matter as long as the chakras connect before you start moving any energy. If you have them sealed and focused before you start running energy, you'll notice the difference. To seal the chakras before working together is a safety issue.

Exercise: How to create a Tantric Field

Here are the instructions for connecting with another human being and creating a vertical Tantric Field. I don't recommend doing this rite with anyone who has no idea what you're doing. Everything you've done so far has brought you to this point, so no one who hasn't done all

> Vertical energy:
> A Tantric field that orients itself with the top and bottom chakras.

that work should try this exercise. The two of you can do this with your clothes on or off, but do it in a sacred, private space. Do not attempt this without the chakra sealing mentioned above.

First, sit down face-to-face, and gaze only into one of your partner's eyes. It's best if you both focus on the right eye, so that you're not tempted to switch glances, which makes your eyes move. Visualize your aura opening up and surrounding the other person like a blanket, and have them do the same. Then open up your chakras as you did in the Flower Bud exercise. Get your partner to do the same. You should be able to feel a psychic "click" happen at this point. If not, look deeply into your partner's eyes, until you can pheel a psychic strangeness. Again, this is experiential, not easy to put into English.

Next, both partners must begin Pranayama breathing in unison. As one partner breathes out, the other partner should be breathing in. Breathe perceptibly to help your partners with their timing. Now, pull the Kundalini up from your base chakra to your crown. If you've been doing your homework, this should only take a few breaths. Once you have the auras wrapped around each other, the chakras connected, the eyes locked, and the breathing synchronized, the Kundalini will naturally want to come up. Now we get to the hard part, which is sharing that energy.

One partner must bring down the Shiva energy, and the other must bring up the Shakti energy. You can choose who does what, but it's easiest for beginning heterosexual males to bring the energy down.

As Shiva energy comes down, it should leap the physical gap between base chakras with no problem; it's going to tend to go there anyway. Shakti energy comes up from the base of the Shakti partner, and goes to Shiva via the crown chakra link. Down Shiva's spine, across the base gap, up Shakti's spine, across the crown gap.

Once this energy has cycled a few times, the couple might get light headed. This is a signal that you have more energy—and oxygen—in your system than your body knows what to do with. You can choose to keep the flow going or end it at that point, or back off.

If you choose to keep the flow going, the light-headedness subsides. The energy in the space between you is a Tantric Field. Be prepared for some intensity in mind, body, and energy, and for the higher vibration to push your life back into balance. The repercussions of pushing yourself beyond your limits are both fascinating and frightening if you're not ready. If you back off from each other or put some object between you, you'll notice that nothing will interrupt the flow short of closing your eyes and willfully backing down, so you must Willfully end it. Respect when your partner signals that he/ she has had enough.

To stop the flow, lean forward and give your partner an embrace, with the intention of "My energy comes back to me, your energy goes back to you." Feel your partner's energy returning to their body, and yours coming back to you. When you feel back to normal again, release the embrace and end the exercise.

How to play safely:

Now think about doing the preceding exercise with someone not nearly as skilled as you are, and then slamming that person with your Kundalini energy. Not only that, but slamming them from the base up. You'd hurt someone. This is why you need to learn to control Kundalini (and Kundalini under sexual stimulation!) to the very nanosecond. Karezza helps, for sure. Recognize, though, that now you have a weapon just as dangerous as a black belt in martial arts, but it's in your sexual response system.

So, how do you practice if you don't have a partner who has clear enough chakras to be safe to work with? Simple; you use nature.

Every waterfall, every tree, every blade of grass is clean, energy wise. Every animal, with the exception of some abused pets, has clear energy you can play with. Every sunrise and sunset has...what? Light. What is light? Energy. What is energy? Stuff that works in your chakras! Hurray!

Exercise: Connecting with Nature

You can open up all your chakras and suck in the sunset while doing Kundalini breathing. Bring it in the crown with the inhale, then exhale, and let it flow back out again through the base. Go hug a tree as you do the flower bud meditation, and then pull in the tree energy through all 7 chakras; exhale and give the tree back some of your energy. Be sure to open up your crown and base chakras, and allow the Shakti energy to enter from below and exit from above, and the Shiva energy from the top down. When you begin moving Kundalini with a partner, you will be bringing the Shiva energy DOWN from above and out the base, into your partner, if you're a male. If you're female, you'll be bringing the Shakti energy up your spine and around the inside of your skull, past your crown and out your third eye. Get used to both flows now.

A few other ways to use nature would be to lie on the earth and breathe with her rhythms, bringing up the serpent in your spine. Go for a bike ride and breathe the wind up to your crown and down to your base. Stand in a circle of maple trees in the fall and breathe in the scent, allowing it to course through your veins as added energy. Many of the things that children do, such as laying on the ground making cloud pictures, spinning in circles looking at the sky, riding bikes, skates and sleds very fast to feel the wind, are instinctive ways that we play with energy as children.

You can feel confident that none of this energy will cause you negative issues. It is "here and now" energy that cannot get 'stuck' in a chakra. Use the memory of these exercises as something beautiful to recall in times of stress.

To work with someone who has "stuck" chakras would cause you all sorts of problems at this point. Think about what energy you would be taking on, if, for example, you connected with someone who was overly paranoid, totally depressed, or had horrible self-esteem or violence issues. No student comes to Tantra with clean energy when beginning work with a guru, but yet the guru must open up to teach such students. This means that it's not impossible, so here's your contemplation:

Question: What is the risk of connecting chakras with people who have major energy problems? How—besides total avoidance—do you protect yourself from that risk, and still connect chakras to someone you want to like/teach/love/have sex with? How do the gurus do it?

That, beloved student, is your puzzle. You will find the answers embedded in later chapters, hidden under innocuous headings. For now, simply contemplate and read on.

Resistance:

Resistance has different meanings in engineering, psychology, and politics. In every case, it means something working against something else.

It has yet another meaning in Tantra. In the pinnacle rite, Maithuna, we're bringing ourselves as close as two people can to becoming the same being, but we are resisting falling completely together. We are holding off from going over the edge into orgasm and actually combining the orgasms. If you put two magnets together with reverse sides and push them as close as you can to each other, one of them tries to flip over and connect, right? They tend to do that naturally. Engineers use this nifty trick to power electric motors. Your job in the Maithuna rite is to keep that resistance, so that you and your partner also become like electromagnets pulling and pushing at the same time.

That's what's difficult to understand from a lot of Tantra books and Eastern-based instruction -- is trying to explain where the energy comes from without delving into mythology. It comes from the resistance; that's all.

Tantrics are being penetrated or penetrating each other's space, becoming one being at the same time. There has to remain an element of withholding, of not letting it combine directly. Because once you do combine the energies, you release them with orgasm, and the Tantric Field backs down to an energetic square one. You are done.

This is why you have to work with the 28-minute touch exercise before getting to this point so you can stay on the edge of that cliff. You can become that polarity magnet with your partner, and build up as much energy as possible before dropping into orgasm, but only if you've got the practice to keep yourself there.

Maithuna must end in orgasm. There's no other way for it to end. But, it's not "just" an orgasm; it is much more. Orgasm is not really a big enough word. It's a very small word for what really happens.

What happens is the energy between the two people gets vibrating higher than what either physical body is capable of doing alone. Therefore, you're going to get to the maximum capacity that your body can handle. You're going to ride that wave as long as possible. At some point, you're going to go over the edge and let your body slip into orgasm. Now the fun thing is that once you connect that tight with your partner, you're not going over the edge alone. It's almost always a mutual orgasm.

As you can imagine, being that closely connected to a partner, if some sort of event happens within their body that is amazing and intense, you're going to have every bit of it slammed into you. Any resistance once someone orgasms is futile. The longer you put that point off, the more energy you will have when you reach the inevitable. Practice with resistance now, utilizing all of the techniques you have learned here, so you can carry that energy for as long as possible.

To resist an orgasm, simply relax, breathe, and be here now. Sounds easy, just like Karezza, right? Get in the habit of this now, so that when you are ready for Maithuna, it becomes second nature.

Horizontal Fields

The horizontal Field is a reinforcement of the vertical field in the exercise above. In creating that field, you put aside all considerations of the individuals creating the field. The Horizontal field is a result of all that the couple is, both sacred and profane.

All that you are with your partner—in this lifetimes and all previous lifetimes—comes into play in creating the Horizontal field.

Begin with a Tantric Field as described in the last section, down one spine and up the next. Then create a ball of energy in each hand of all that you have shared together as friends, partners, or lovers. All of your history and all of your future are in your hands. Next, link hands as well as all other linkages going on with the original field. Allow the energy to circulate in a clockwise fashion through your heart chakras and your palm chakras. You will find the Horizontal field manifesting after a few short cycles

What does this do for you? Primarily it creates a more intense healing field than the first exercise. Anything placed in this field will change—even some non-living things. It also creates a connection between working partners that allows them to vibrate higher than any other energy in the vicinity. This allows them to work on larger projects such as clearing buildings of negativity, ridding people of ghosts and other following energies, giving energy to volunteerism, and cutting unhealthy connections for others. In other words, it allows a Priest or Priestess to operate as clergy for their community as well.

Once the couple tunes in to each other both vertically and horizontally, they may find that they can actually even feel each other's skin sensations to a certain degree. One of the more advanced Tantric exercises is to facilitate that experience intentionally. Create the connection with a partner, and then take turns feeling each other's touches. This makes for a very interesting experiment, and if your partner is your lover, it could lead to some very odd experiences during ordinary sex, as you can now feel exactly what you are doing to your partner. This is experiential--English can never really cover it correctly.

Another good experiment for couples is to put distance between them after creating the Horizontal field, and see how large they can

> Horizontal energy:
> Energy shared via the heart chakra and palm chakras. Usually this energy involves the sum total of what the two can be to each other.

make the field grow between them. The larger the field, the larger the work they can accomplish. Usually, a full-length room is a good enough distance to heal anything that needs healing.

Reverse Polarity

One of the exercises I insist that a student be proficient in is what I refer to as "Reverse Polarity." Most energy we experience with our base chakras is going out the male's base chakra and coming into the female's base chakra. This is typical, and the return of the energy exits the female through the eyes via the crown chakra, enters the male body via his eyes, then his crown chakra and back down his spine. However, with reverse polarity, you do just the opposite; you send base chakra energy from the female's yoni to the male's lingam, bring that vibration up the male spine and out the male crown chakra, back to the acceptant female eyes and crown chakra, and then down the female spine. Same thing you have been doing, only backwards.

The trick to this reverse of polarity is that the male must intentionally open the base chakra and relax the muscles that habitually tense up at his groin. The female must open channels in her scalp and neck muscles to accommodate the incoming energy. The Pranayama breathing remains the same, just the focus changes. You can do this by intentional mental manipulation of the aura and clearing of the chakras with the tools given earlier.

Negativity:

As a Tantric, you will come to know when you're in need of balance, and when you are carrying someone else's blocks, or when you are free and clear of all programs. Something within you will stop you and say, "This is not my issue." If you can trace the beginning of any weird feeling back to it's source in time, and you find that it began manifesting after an intimate moment with someone else, and that someone else has blocks you know about, you can be pretty sure you've taken on their transferred issue.

How is that possible? As Einstein says, energy and matter are interchangeable, depending on the speed of the object. Energy that is vibrating slower will have a more physical pheel to it. You can test this out by taking note of your body's reaction when you think of happy thoughts or depressive thoughts. No one who thinks of depressing thoughts will feel as if weight has LEFT them in a test like this. This is because emotional energy does have weight and mass to it. Simply because scientists have not developed machines to measure it does not mean it weighs nothing.

The other thing we know from science is that emotions left to fester in our subconscious will create negative behavior patterns. If left alone long enough, these patterns become solids, with as much weight and mass as any energy form could possibly acquire. When you examine your Abyss issues, you are dealing with this type of construct directly. When left alone, however, these constructs create a pocket of negative energy that begins to take on a life of it's own. It tends to follow around its creator, leading to more and more negativity piling onto it, as well as into its creator's environment. We call these constructs emotional baggage, vampires, demons, and gremlins in other cultures; simply naming them is giving them energy, so we refer to them vaguely.

People who are chronically depressed tend to have this sort of 'black cloud' energy hanging around them, as do people who are chronically addicted to substances or gambling. The rule to remember is this: If you got it from someone else, it should go away with grounding. If, however, it was something you created yourself, the only way to get rid of it is to walk through the Abyss that created it and dump the energy.

Working with untrained people:

In a perfect world, we would all have our partners beside us from the beginning of Tantric training. It would be someone we love who would be willing to learn this path beside us, to follow the pitfalls with us, to emerge at the end as a suitable partner for Maithuna.

I have yet to meet anyone who lived in that world. Many people learn Tantra solo and take it back to their partner, or wait until they find a partner, and try to share the interest. Sometimes two trained Tantrics will meet and create a relationship that includes Tantra, but that is the most rare of occurrences.

For the most part, however, trained Tantrics find themselves having sex with untrained partners, and keeping their Tantric practice out of the bedroom. This is not a necessary turn of events for all students. It is possible to practice Tantra on a mild scale with a partner who has no previous training in Tantra.

There are a few things to be cautious of, though. First, it really is best to you're your lovers know that you study Tantra, if that's possible, in conversation before heading to the bedroom. Sometime between the first kiss and the first piece of clothing off, you should find a moment to say, "Have you ever heard of Tantra?" and let the conversation lead from there.

Secondly, never take your vibration to maximum capacity power with someone who is not ready. If you want to heal this person, you should be prepared to go the distance with them through the process. Because you will raise their vibration. Whatever is wrong with their energy will self-correct, and that's not always pleasant, nor understandable. Unless you are a professional psychologist, avoid that issue all together by practicing at lower vibrational levels with an untrained partner, or not at all.

The puppy-dog effect

It is possible that you give an untrained lover a craving for your energy that they cannot explain or are not equipped to deal with. This could manifest as stalking and harassment. When doing Tantra with untrained individuals, you run the risk of them attributing the great sex to your personal prowess. They become like a puppy-dog, following you around, waiting for the next chance to have sex with you.

Even if you're normally vibrating everyday at a higher rate than most people are, you can really shock people's systems, not always in a good way. If somebody is receiving more energy than they're putting out, you're risking the puppy dog effect. If you have fantastic sex with another person who is not capable of doing the energetic work that you're doing, it's liable to be the best sex they ever had, even if you didn't consider it unusually grand.

Suddenly they're following you around, or messing with your energy every chance they get. If they can't turn you on, they try to piss you off...anything to get you to pay attention to them. Be aware that if you get into a sexual situation with someone who is not vibrating very high and you bring your vibration up they're going to find it very fun and very tasty and very attractive. It can be like an addiction. You're helping them reach mindsets they've never had. To them it's something that they didn't do for themselves. It came from another source—YOU. To their perspective, you must be the thing that they need.

When a person raises energy and vibration, what happens when they have unresolved issues and blocks? They will start coming into balance and shaking off their old habits and baggage, which will reflect in their environment, which will become forced changes.

Remember all the hard work that you went thru when you were walking thru the Abyss? You can set this off in other people by merely raising their vibration. Since they haven't learned to sustain that vibration, how to ground, or even how to get out of the Abyss again, this could be dangerous. They don't have a way to figure out what is going on as a Tantric student would. They don't know about wallowing through the Abyss, or body memory, or reprogramming.

They could be in for a real rough time with lots of issues. They might get back into one of their past issues and not come out again, running off with the first thing that walks in the room, selling their house, or quitting a lifetime career.

Tantra expedites processing your baggage. Anyone you affect with it has to deal with his or her own issues anyway. They can't just run away from it, because it's a part of them. To do that to somebody who is not aware that it can even happen is, well...that's just plain mean.

You now have the responsibility for your energy. You know what's going on; you know what you can do. It is your responsibility where and when you use it. If you're not willing to help that person heal, don't get into higher vibrations with them. Tantra is not a good thing to pull out on a one-night stand.

> ## A confidence boost:
>
> Sometimes a student takes his or her newfound talents into the world to show off. Student "B" found himself suddenly dealing with his partner's issues this way. He met a young lady who was coming out of an addiction and a bad relationship at the same time. They had sex, and both of them came to me talking about how great the sex was. They looked like two people in love. About two days later, she was feeling empowered and went to her ex's house, confrontationally, and was severely battered by her still-addicted ex boyfriend. B felt responsible for it because he knew he had temporarily empowered her, but he wasn't acting responsible at the time, he was just having fun. He had no idea that her newfound confidence would get her in that much trouble.
>
> B wound up taking her under his wing, moving her into his house, and then realizing that she was not ready to heal. The connection was not real love; it was just a vibration thing. He slowed down his own progress because his energy got taken up by a needy partner who needed him to help her thru what he helped push her into. This behavior led to a lot of stormy short-lived relationships for him, and his life was not very happy until he recognized it as his own Karma many years later.

A self-regulating field.

There are no such things as "evil" Tantrics. It will let you try your limit. It will let you put energy into things that might seem negative, but the repercussions and manifestations of that are also negative. Any action of ill intent will come right back at you. This could do anything necessary for your Karma to help you to heal from whatever caused you to have an ill purpose in the first place.

In that way, it really is self-regulating. You can screw up once but then you fix it, learn from it, and don't do it again. You WILL manifest something when you use the energies. What ever is going on in your head when you orgasm will become part of your life. There's no way of getting it to stop at that point. Many people may laugh at this concept, but a few self-experiments usually change that attitude.

Even if the thought is "let's do this again," it will manifest. When the ill intent is there, or the unawareness, or the unawareness of the partner, or the unawareness of our own baggage, you begin manifesting strong life lessons. There's no good and bad, it's a matter of how you deal with it.

Orgasm Power!

Resistance is the opposite of surrender. When we bring our energy level up to the edge of the cliff and hang there, we are practicing Resistance Tantra. The point of this is to build energy up for higher vibrational meditations. When we relax and allow ourselves to slip into repeated orgasms, giving in to the feelings in our bodies, we call this 'surrender' Tantra. It is not possible to practice both resistance and surrender at the same time, however, it is important to learn the difference and to master one before approaching the other.

I insist that my students learn to resist before they learn to surrender. When working with surrender Tantra, keep in mind how an orgasm travels in waves. Like a pebble in a pond, it moves out from its source, affecting the energy around it in waves of high vibration. In ordinary lovemaking, this is what creates a deep connection between lovers. This is what also creates thick connectivity between orgy participants. Orgasm creates an environment where even shallow connections can become semi-permanent.

When a Tantric has Kundalini energy at maximum capacity power and then releases the energy in orgasm, anyone and everyone in the room is going to feel it and be aware of the energy explosion. Sometimes even people in the next room will feel it. Untrained individuals will find themselves inexplicably tied to the orgasmic person, and a link can form inadvertently. When either partner in a couple with Tantric energy in their systems has an orgasm, it creates a strong connective link between them that gives them more psychic ability than normal.

It doesn't even matter where the bodies are in relation to each other. I've seen instances where orgasmic energy has affected people over 15 feet away from each other with walls in between. Intense orgasmic energy will linger in the physical realm sometimes, which is why adult arcades and porn stores have a peculiar pheeling to them that keeps many people away.

Orgasms fueled by Kundalini, Karezza, and resistance are more energetic than any other type. This type of orgasm will raise the vibration of anyone exposed to the energy, and subsequently force the energy into healthier patterns. The degree of force upon their energy is in direct relation to the amount of energy the couple is capable of raising. Nevertheless, forcefully raising someone else's vibration is not a good idea. Learning to control your own orgasmic energy, especially with raised vibrations, is important to your own safety and the safety of others.

Some may think deprivation or celibacy exercises are old

> Deprivation:
> To keep yourself away from an item or substance. Excess: Doing too much of something. The opposite of deprivation.

fashioned, but celibacy and fasting are practices that can help you learn the skills of resistance. Resistance, indeed, is a skill. All chakras have a need that fills them, and reducing or removing that need helps you discover what it takes to resist energy in general. Go back to Chapter 2, and think about the information offered there.

Groundwork:

White: Making love to yourself (described earlier)

Red: Resistance Vs. Surrender: Sit facing one another, holding hands. Recognize what this does to the energy between you. See if you find yourself drawn to or pushed away from this person's energy. Now move your faces close, keeping your noses about two inches apart. See if you are able to control what your eyes and breath are doing. Keep breathing in a relaxed manner, falling back into Pranayama if you can. Gaze into your partner's eyes; is this pulling you in or pushing you away?

Now move even closer to your partner, as if you were going to kiss, but stop an inch from touching lips. Control your breathing still; keep your eyes open still. Focus on the sensations in your body.

The act of stopping at this point creates resistance in your system. That resistance, when left to it's own devices, will either pull you in toward the kiss or push you away from the kiss, depending on your intentions toward your partner (and your partner's intention toward you!). Doing NOTHING about the situation--i.e. neither going forward into the kiss nor allowing the energy to make you back up—is the only way to create the tension in your body known as resistance, which is another good way to increase the available amount of electricity in your neurons.

Hold that resistance position as long as you can. Relax and breathe into it, allowing the tension to run through all your body parts, much like in the Karezza exercise, and then out your limbs. When you finally give into the pull or push, pay attention to the amount of energy in your system when you release the tension. Compare this resistance energy to the energy of Karezza.

Blue: Community Weaving Rite:

Have a common goal in mind, such as building something new, or healing a particular person, place, or situation. This ritual will create a connection between community members on a Heart Chakra level in perfect love and perfect trust. Partners should be across from each other to gaze into each other's eyes. Connect with the people in the room as best as possible before sitting down into circle. When you are finally all seated facing each other, drop shields & masks, connect with the eyes of every person in the circle.

Have everyone connect with Shiva and Shakti, putting roots down into the ground, and branches into the sky. Allow them to meld and circulate together. Placing the right hand on the front of the heart chakra of the person next to you, place your left hand on the person's back, at the heart chakra to the left of you. Overlap hands. All of you connect to four other people. Bring energy from your right to your left, through your heart chakra.

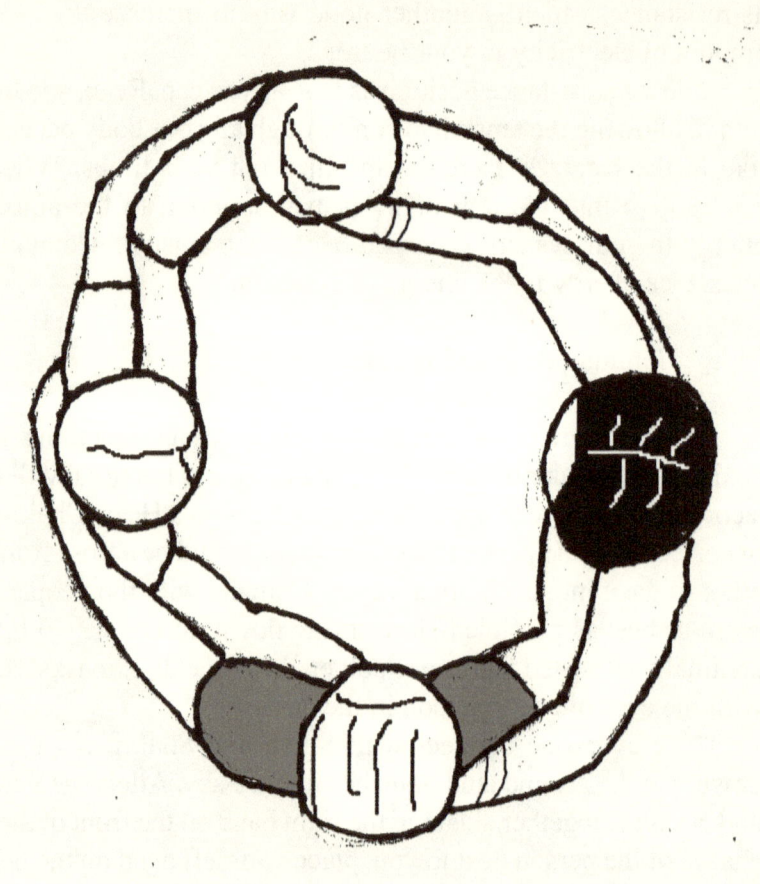

Group connecting

Breathing alternately with half of the circle, using a 4:4 beat, practice by exhaling smoothly, inhaling smoothly, exhaling smoothly. Count off around the circle, Red/Blue or 1's and 2's. The Reds should exhale and the Blues should inhale with some cue, and then the Reds should inhale and the Blues exhale simultaneously as well. A drummer or metronome works well for the signals for this.

Allow this breathing pattern to continue until people attain a meditative headspace. At that point, everyone can begin describing his or her visions verbally. As you exhale, speak a few words of what you are seeing. Do not attempt to speak while inhaling. Listen and make an effort to see what they are seeing.

Don't let conflicting visions keep you from speaking what you are seeing.

These may simply be decisions that are not yet made. When the words of description have come to a slow, begin with a hum or "om." You may sing a constant tone, or chant your own mantra. Allow the energy of the group to build. Visualize yourself building a path of your choice, coming from that vision and leading back to the here & now.

See your brothers and sisters here helping you build the path. Try to harmonize your humming tone with those of the people around you; take this tone and use it as your building tools for the path. Allow the noise/hum/om to end as naturally as it wants to. Allow all minds to float on this higher vibration into the astral realms.

Let go of your brothers and sisters, lay back on the floor, and let everyone space out. The group should now be something akin to a carpet of bodies on the floor. Ask yourself "what is my part in this work?" The floating should allow you to find a clue.

If you must, bring everyone back with a gentle reminder to return to this reality. You will know they are back when all sitting up again. Release any residual energy into the ground.

Chapter 8:   The Puja

Puja worship history & reasons

What separates Red Tantra from all other forms of spirituality, meditation, yoga, or worship is that Red Tantra is for two people. It is the only inner spiritual practice designed to share.

One of the high points of shifting from White Tantra to Red Tantra is the inclusion of the Shiva-Shakti Puja ritual. Maithuna is the most honored and respectful thing you can do as a couple. The Shiva-Shakti Puja is the most honored and respectful path of to get from White Tantra to Red Tantra. This Puja ritual has been called "pink Tantra" for it's purpose as a segue between White Tantra and Red Tantra.

The word "Puja" means "worship." There are Pujas done to all Hindu gods and goddesses, but the Tantric Shiva-Shakti puja teaches you to worship your lover —and allow your lover to worship you. It starts with a ritualized version of the chakra sealing mentioned before, and it ends with recognition of the partner as Divine. The Bhakti work you did in the Heart Cave was only a step in this direction. Now you

> Puja:
> A particular ritual done by two people as an introduction to higher Tantric rites. Puja usually includes compliments, honoring, and gifting.

must open up to allow another human being to worship the Naked Flame inside of you, and you must endeavor to do the same in return. Approach this as you would any important date.

The couple must do this ritual in sacred space. Ritual bathing before getting into the ritual, and uses of perfumes & oils are all traditional ways to please the partner and recognize this event as a unique and special occurrence. Makeup, jewelry, clothing, and body paint are all appropriate ways of decorating yourself as a figure of worship.

The temple itself should be set up with pillows and soft spaces to sit. Also, all of the equipment you will be using should be within easy reach of where you intend to sit. Have plenty of drinking water within reach, as this ritual will increase body temperature and thirst.

American Pujas:

Many groups I've encountered host what they call "Puja rituals." They differ in scope and action by a large margin, with very little in common from one to the next. In most public Pujas in America, there is a theme of Bhakti, or Worship. Either a single Deity depicted on an altar, or a live human being, in the form of one's partner, is the item worshipped. Some Pujas require a circle of men and a circle of women to face each other during the worship. Some pujas require that everyone circle around the center altar.

Shiva-Shakti Pujas are "Adult" rituals. It's not adult rated because of nudity, but because of the energy moving around. The content of the energy is highly erotic, as energy goes. The really cool thing about American Tantra is that we can get beyond doing Pujas in any specific way. You are free to make it your own ritual. Those things are all up to you. The important thing is to acknowledge each chakra, and as partners, open up those chakras entirely.

My method for this ritual is to invoke both God and Goddess into a one of each partner, and worship each other. We share the Sacred Couple's romantic energies with each other and subsequently with everyone and everything else in the room in the form of gifts like poetry, incense, wine, flowers, chocolate, etc. Then we take all that heavy infused romantic flirty lustful energy, and, depending on the group, either allow it to play out, or allow the attendees to take it home.

The traditional Shiva-Shakti Puja ritual is actually a Pre-ritual ritual. It's the ritual that you do before you do the REAL Tantric ritual, which is where penetration actually happens and Maithuna begins. This Puja is a way for the couple to get their energy levels matched together before going into the bedroom and getting involved in Sacred Sex. As such, the end of the Shiva-Shakti Puja is not written...makes sense! Every time you do it, it ends in a different way.

My High Priest and I have done this ritual over a dozen times in various settings. We've had great rituals each time, but each ending had it's own personality. Some times, it turns into a very large and happy orgy, or every couple for themselves having sex in corners leaving the big spaces open. Sometimes it turns into heavy drinking and singing sailor songs, and nobody gets naked at all. Sometimes everyone leaves except two or three people who stay and eat strawberries and cream all night. Sometimes it turns into a deep discussion of occult theory between eight people of the same gender. I've seen puppy piles, one-on-one teacher/student relations, tarot readings, champagne proposals, and all sorts of loving, caring activity come down after puja. Anything goes, as long as it's relaxing, it feels good and is mutually happy for all.

Physical side effects

When practicing any sort of Red Tantra you should know that there will be a lot more sexual fluids than you are accustomed to. If you allow yourself an orgasm either during or after connecting with another person in a Tantric field, you will find that there is a lot of female ejaculate, a copious amount of ejaculation in males, and a lot of multiple orgasms in both.

Also, the gender traits become less specific, because you're blending the balance of both people. We lose the physical body and we lose all the things we are normally aware of during sex, like the bed, the scent of the air, or the lighting in the room. All these things are no longer a factor. Even if you are releasing your own resistance energy through Karezza, you'll have these extra fluids and this loss of reality.

This is why Tantric sex is possible between same-sex couples. Shiva and Shakti are in everything, and should exist in all people in equal amounts. We loose everything at the moment of orgasm, so therefore, it doesn't matter what gender you or your partner are.

All thoughts of identity, even the questions of whether or not you are doing it right, disappear in the moment of orgasm. As you recognize the Divine in your partner, recognize that you're also bringing Divinity into your body. You're no longer two people having sex. These are deities coming together. Granted, using your physical bodies is necessary to get there, but you forget about them once you get into that space where nothing else matters, where there is no Time.

Once you are in that space and can achieve that, you're able to carry more energy every other moment of your life, even when you're not with your partner having sex or doing Maithuna or pujas. You don't slide back to your beginning state; you do come down, but relative to where you were. You never come down to the state you were before you started.

You will notice that you have more energy in daily life once you've done the Maithuna rite. Of course, Maithuna is not a finite action either. Just because you've done it once, it was fantastic, and you got there doesn't mean you can't do it again. Each time will be different.

We can't, of course, do Maithuna every day, even though many of us want to. There's a lot of preparation and you have to do it with great intent and purpose. You will find that it is well worth it. All other sex will pale in comparison.

That doesn't mean you can't just have quickies, or just go out and get laid, or even just have ordinary sex, you just kinda, well...you don't want to. It will always remind you of the possibilities of what you could be doing. You can, however, incorporate the Tantric field every time if you have a long-term relationship. My partner and I joke that we have forgotten how to have "regular" sex. It's not that we've forgotten 'how'...we've simply forgotten 'why' when we can have Tantric sex every time.

Why do the puja at all?

Shivashakti Puja requires that we acknowledge and honor each chakra. For every chakra, touch it and say something about your partner that you admire. Speak from the heart, give from the heart, and be real about it. If you don't personalize it, it's not going to mean as much, and it's not going to stick in your head. Once you're into Maithuna, you're not going to recall what it was that you did. When you do something from the heart, with meaning, it gives you a wedge against going over the cliff into orgasm. If you're doing Maithuna, and you get to the point where you're fighting the resistance, the magnetism will pull you closer. If you don't recognize that this person in front of you is the Divine energy, what you see when you look at that person is your ordinary lover, someone you are used to filling up with your energy all the time. So, you say to yourself "Why not now?"

And then what? You just want to jump their bones; you just want to have rockin' sex. That's the intensity you're dealing with. If you do a Shivashakti Puja before Maithuna, it helps to hold you in that state, anchored in the Inner Self, reminding you what you're doing here. It allows the Inner mind to get the message across to your conscious mind that "This is something different." It will keep you from just falling into that "gotta have it" mentality.

Yes, it is no myth that Tantrics stay coupled for hours on end, with no loss of erection, no loss of lubrication, nobody gets worn out, and nobody gets sore. It's about the energy moving from one set of chakras to another, then back again, like a flywheel in an electric motor. It's not about how fast a lingam can pump in and out of a yoni. If the chakras are sealed and the energy is flowing, no bodies need to pump anything. That's how Tantrics have sex for impossible-seeming durations. Doing the puja before doing Maithuna makes this possible.

To participate in Maithuna requires both partners to have the ability to keep Kundalini energy running, be fully invoked of Shiva or Shakti energy, and also to be able to stay sexually stimulated and aroused without going over the edge of the cliff for the duration of the rite. How long is the rite? Well, as you may know by now, the moment that one or the other participants goes into orgasm, the game is over, the fun has ended. Pack up your toys and go home.

Puja forms: White Tantra (solo)

The term Siddhaka signifies an image of the deity. (When doing double puja, the Siddhaka is a live person). This image can be a picture, an object that reminds you of your personal connection to that deity, or a statue of that deity. Statues take more wear and tear than anything else, and therefore are the most popular for use in puja.

Set up the altar with candles, incense, three flowers, a water pitcher and chalice, a wine bottle and chalice, different food gifts like chocolate and grapes, and a mandala or other device to represent the visual aspect of the deity. When using Siddhaka, it should be separate from all these other elements on the altar, perhaps in the center of it all, or in front of the other items. Or, if very large, beside the altar, with the Siddhaka on the right and the altar on the left.

Once the altar is set up, sit lotus style in front of the altar. Speak the words out loud, with feeling, as if you were actually speaking to the Deity him/herself. Don't read out loud from what is written here; use this as a guide to write your own lines that will mean more to you. You may sing the chants at the end if music is what you hear when you speak them.

Exercise: Shiva Puja

Speak these words to your Siddhaka:

> *"Oh Lord Shiva, who art Vishnu, who art Brahma, who art Matter, who art Light, who are the Sun, who art physical being in all it's created forms.*

> *(Light Candles, hold up to Siddhaka in toast.)*

> *"Shiva, my master, who is Father, Brother, Son and Lover. You are divine, and I am a humble mortal in your presence.*

> *(Light Incense, hold up to Siddhaka to smell.)*

> *"I thank you for your graciousness, in all that manifests in our universe. Your gift to humanity is a boon and we are grateful.*

> *(offer one flower to the Altar, or placed at Siddhaka feet.*

> *"You provide the form and the substance for all of Creation, and our appreciation*

> *reaches to the depths of our beings.*

> *(Pour water into chalice and raise glass to Siddhaka*

"I give to you this mortal frame, to take as yours, to become one with mankind.

Take this opportunity, oh mighty Shiva, to experience this (flesh and blood)

physical body.

(Pinch rice from bowl & sprinkle on Siddhaka's feet.)

"I long to see your face, to hear your voice to touch your skin. I long to show you my love and appreciation for your grace.

(Pour wine from bottle into chalice and pour then raise in front of

Siddhaka)

"Use this human form to recall how all that is male is part of you, but also how he has learned to serve you.

(Pinch food from platter and place on altar, then on ground in front of

Siddhaka)

"Allow your presence to manifest upon this human body, as a gift and a sacrifice to you, my beautiful Lord Shiva.

(kiss Siddhaka)

"Om Namah Shiva, Om."

Shakti puja:

(follow ritual above, changing only the wording. The triple aspects

of Shakti are Parvati, Saraswati, and Kali. All gift correspondences remain the same.)

Double Puja--Red Tantra

This Shiva-Shakti Puja ritual was experimental, in that the ritual did not come to me in this format, nor can I recall the actual source. Probably it came from an undocumented (and probably plagarized) website. With this information, I went into meditation and was "shown" this ritual on a different level. What I present below is a creation that is partially mine, partially divinely inspired, and partially from another forgotten source. After over a dozen public performances of this ritual with my High Priest, I have yet to have an unsatisfactory experience with it. The format is impressive within a community setting, and is an excellent "blue" Tantra exercise for a group.

To do Shivashakti puja means to bring both Shiva and Shakti into two physical bodies, and allow them to carry out their duties as divine couple on the physical plane, whatever those duties are. This is a "red Tantra" ritual in that it takes two people to execute. To set up this ritual takes at least 3 days, but is most successful if carried thru an entire moon cycle (28 days).

Both participants should work simultaneously but in separate locations until the actual ritual. During this setup time, each participant should be doing daily separate pujas to Shiva and to Shakti. The Priest who is going to embody Shiva during the actual ceremony should become familiar with Shakti as a lover during this time. The Priestess who will embody Shakti should be training herself as Shiva's lover. (Gender pronouns really mean nothing here; either deity can be embodied or become the lover of either male or female.)

See the previous puja exercise for how to do a solo White puja. When calling upon the God or Goddess, remember that you must also be an attractive beacon for him/her to appear. Realize that Shiva is always attracted to Shakti, and she is always attracted to Him. Contemplate that she is Energy, he is Matter. Astrally make love to the deities when they appear in your visualizations or meditations. Actively allow either of them to manifest for a short while within your physical system. Make them part of your daily life during this pre-puja setup time.

Ritual Steps

The humans who are prepared to receive deity must be in meditative state during the ritual. Each person is now the Siddhaka to the other. For best results, they should have not had harsh chemicals in their system in 7 days (prescription or recreational drugs, medical treatments, environmental hazards), sex in 3 days, food in one day and water in three hours. For best results, this Siddhaka should have Kundalini activated for this rite, and both participants should be nude.

Since we invoke both Shiva and Shakti, the ritual simultaneously honors Shiva first, then Shakti, then Shiva, etc. The actual order of who goes first does not matter. Set up the altar with candles, incense, flowers (6 for dual rites), a water pitcher and 2 chalices, two bottles of wine, red and white, and a chalice for each, green and red grapes, and two plates of chocolate. You can swap these gifts for anything you like; we have used anointing oils, peacock feathers, rice, meat, fish, and all sorts of other edibles.

Make sure your altar also contains a bell, and a mandala to represent the visual aspect of the deity. A ritual foot washing with sandalwood scent (male first) and chakra sealing (male first) can precede all. The couple should have a pillow on which to sit during the rite, with the Priestess sitting on the lap of the Priest, who is sitting on the pillow. The couple should sit in yabyum position, with Kundalini aroused and chakras connected throughout the whole rite (see Maithuna in chapter 9 for more descriptions on this).

This is a ritual of love, of flirting, of romance and play, designed to lead directly into sex upon completion. Feed lines to each other designed to tantalize the participants as well as each other. As Shiva and Shakti share gifts to honor each other, share the gifts with all of the

> **Yab yum:**
> A position that a couple takes when practicing Red Tantra. This position has one partner sitting in the lap of another.

participants in the ritual. Pass the food and drink to the others in the circle, with the help of assistants if necessary. These gifts can be coordinated with your chakras. Remind the participants that as they pass the gifts to the person beside them that he or she is also an embodiment of Shiva or Shakti, and that they are honoring the chakra energy in this person as well as allowing their own energy to be honored.

In the end you may chant, males with Shiva, females with Shakti. The chant is "Om Namah Shiva Om" or "Om Namah Shakti Om." Namah means "Great, fantastic, fabulous." Therefore, Om Namah Shakti Om, means, "Fabulous is the goddess Shakti!" You can do these separately or overlap them in creative ways unique to your style. Encourage the attendees to chant with you, so you can share in the Joy of their Creating Shivashakti, the apex of Matter meeting Energy, Sky meeting Earth, Male meeting Female. The final chant of their coming together is "Om Namah Shivashakti Om".

During the chanting phase, focus on bringing up Kundalini energy to maximum capacity power. The Tantric field thus created expands outward to encompass all participants in the ritual. After signalling the end of the chanting, both Priest and Priestess should allow their consciousness to release and the Deities to manifest. At this point, any magicks that the couple deem suitable for God and Goddess to participate in should take place. This includes sexual union in Maithuna, orgasmic energy release for sex magick, and any more mundane projects.

Altar checklist:
2 of everything:
Chalices for water
Chalices for wine
Water bottles
Wine bottles (white shiva, red Shakti)
Chocolate (broken into bite sizes)
Candles (white shiva, red shakti)
Incense
Anointing oils
Grapes (white shiva, red Shakti)
Shivashakti statue

IMPORTANT: *Both priest and priestess must be well versed in resistance Tantra, or else the puja will end abruptly with the couple copulating rather than meditating. Neither Priest nor Priestess should allow any sexual release before the end of the puja, or it my skew the energy of the group..*

Americans can bend this ritual in any way that they feel will work best, and they can end it any way as well. (The ancient Tantrics didn't have chocolate to work with!) The end of the double puja is unwritten, as it should always be. It is the ritual before Maithuna, and therefore should never be scripted. If the couple so chooses to surrender to the energy of the puja, the result will be a phenomenal release of energy at the end, suitable for self-enlightenment, self-healing, and major vibrational shifts. If they choose to direct that energy into more physically oriented projects, both should release their energy in separate ways so as not to overload their own karmic systems.

Instant Healing (Sienna's story)

As I was writing this book, I took a fall while camping and seriously injured my back. I was flat on my back for a month...a month leading up to a scheduled public Puja ritual. At this time, no one else in the local community had the training to take my place. With painkillers out of the question, I decided that perhaps a puja would help heal the problem.

My High Priest and I were very accustomed to each other's energy, and as we sat in Yabyum position, he was careful to help me get comfortable on a pillow between his knees before we began exchanging energy. We circulated energy for about three breaths when strange music from outside distracted us for a moment.

I took that opportunity to stretch out backwards one more time before the crowd would be entering the temple. As I lay backwards across the floor of the temple, my pelvis still higher up on the pillow, my legs stretched around my partner, there was an audible "pop!" in the joint I had injured. Both of us heard it. The relief from the pain was instantaneous!

A look of concern crossed the Priest's face for just a moment, before he realized that the "pop" was relief and not more injury. We both recognized that the three small breaths we had circulated were already putting my energy back where it belonged. By the time the crowd entered the temple, my back felt better than it had in a month. By the end of the puja, almost all of the pain had subsided, and we had a wonderful Temple night.

Groundwork:

White: solo puja (described earlier)

Red: Creating the Tantric Field (described earlier)

Blue: Public Puja as described earlier.

Chapter 9:　Maithuna

The Climax:

Maithuna is the climax of Tantric practices. I will not call it the "climax of Tantra" because that is a personal and individualized Tantric experience, however, the ritual aspect of Left-handed Red Tantra focuses on the rite of Maithuna.

Maithuna is the combination of the Shiva and Shakti force on a physical level. It is the one ritual where Male and Female physical generative organs come together while the mental and spiritual aspects of Shiva and Shakti fuse as well. Maithuna IS the penetrative sexual aspect of Tantra.

Maithuna is not merely a matter of having sex, because the energies of Shiva and Shakti must be flowing in both Priest and Priestess. It is not merely a matter of spiritual invocation, because the physical lingam goes into the physical yoni and both partners must withhold typical orgasm, usually for hours on end. To conquer both the physical restraint and the energetic surrender aspects of Maithuna requires expertise in everything you've done so far.

Karma:

The moment you began practicing Pranayama, you began clearing up your own energy. That kicked off a process which helped you feel healthier, and gave you resolve to go on to the next exercise. No matter where you are now in your practice, you are in the process of clearing your energy. However, to accomplish Maithuna, your chakras must be functional to the point of being able to recognize your own Karma when you see it.

What is your own Karma? It's when your actions have negative repercussions on the physical plane that get out of your control. We don't have to worry about Karma incurred before this lifetime; we can create enough for ourselves in an ordinary lifespan to keep us busy. Recognizing our Karma is a skill that keeps us from making the same mistakes twice, and allows us to correct the trajectory of events before they happen. To do this, you have to have clear flowing energy.

Clear flowing energy allows us to catch all the details in any situation. With clear chakras, we interpret events without emotional overtones, staying focused in the present. This gives us more information than the average guy gets, which gives us better decision making capabilities, which allows us to not create problems for ourselves. Ta da! Automatic clear Karma.

It truly is self-regulating. It's a skill that you learn, like hitting a home run. Pay attention to what's going on around you. Figure out what your emotional reactions are, and start 'acting' rather than 'reacting'. Get therapy if you need it. Paying attention to your good days and bad days will give an idea of what your own patterns are, of what works for you and what doesn't. Play into the patterns actively instead of trying to change them reactively; this will help you learn where you're path is leading you.

Reading situations, living at higher vibrational rates, and continuing to clear your energy gives you an awareness of local energetic subtleties. It means that you're aware of who is in the room, what their energy is doing, and how you're going to react when you encounter them.

When you're aware of your own energy and how that relates to the world around you, it's apparent that other people are acting as a result of the energy around them, too. Though it may be entirely unconscious to them, you have the insight of what their chakras are doing and why you react the way you do. All of these energies are always there; you are now learning to use them to your advantage.

Once you begin living life through the experiences of Tantra, it's difficult to go back from that to a lesser vibrational state, although it is possible. You can close off those insights, ignore your best instincts, close the door on good habits, change your diet for the worse and you will be back down where you were. That level will always be there. But, keep in mind that there will always be the knowledge that you have already gained.

Love and the Chakras

Love is the most powerful force in the universe; however, most of us do not know what it means to love. Some have come to believe that love is a myth, a fantasy not attainable in this loveless society. Some think that love will save them from themselves. Many people define love as "the commitment, respect, and concern for a person's growth." That person could be the self, or it could be the beloved. This could be said of romantic relationships as well as parent/child relationships. Loving is a conscious, Willful act.

Love must be given to be received. In Red Tantra, we must offer Love from all seven chakras to the beloved. You must be able to love their mind, their words, their heart, their environment, their habits, and their sexuality. If you cannot allow yourself to open up to another person, entirely, you will not be successful with Maithuna. This means to connect and share energy with them on every level. If your partner is not trustworthy on any of those levels, then the ability to be entirely open is lost. You cannot have a balanced sending or receiving of Red Tantric energy if one person is holding back.

To work with a partner, all communications should be toward positive ends that foster self-esteem in the other. Gossip and lies do not further anyone's growth, so Tantric practitioners shun these activities. Threats and violence are absolutely not acceptable methods of communication. If it doesn't make you feel good when you walk away, it wasn't healthy.

If all communications came from a space of true love, where we actually cared about growth, it would change the human condition. Since we can't change other people, we can change ourselves. Do everything you can to foster growth in other living things, and you will find that your energy comes back to you 10 fold. If you find you cannot love someone entirely, figure out why. It's not about them; it's about your ability to love. There should be nothing to fear in love.

Civilized Sex:

When you watch any Maithuna ritual, from the outside, it doesn't look like much is happening. Some movie producers once contacted me to make a "Tantric porn" movie. They were a little frustrated when I told them it doesn't make good porn. There is no real visible movement. Yes, the lingam is nice and snug inside the yoni, but nobody's moving. Because there's no movement necessary. The only thing that's moving is the lingam and the yoni themselves, hidden from view. And, the energy that is moving thru the two humans with their breaths. Not much to film, eh?

Tantra is not a spectator sport. It is not fun to watch, although the two people moving the energy between them are having the time of their life. Internally, it's very intense, but from an outside perspective...

It looks very boring.

Especially to a culture that bases its sexuality on visuals, pornography, wild movements, and focus on body parts. People expecting to see some fantastic feats of sexuality are going to be highly disappointed watching a Maithuna rite, unless

> **Contraction:**
> A shudder or shiver that runs through your body that culminates in your genital muscles.

they are participants. It's really not about getting off, and it's not about being sexy. It's about the experience, the connection, the energy, the intensity, the cycle, and the vortex of energy created by Maithuna.

This is how Tantrics can get away with actually having sex for hours and hours. It's not a myth. Yet, they're not wearing themselves out trying to screw like rabbits having orgasm after orgasm. As a matter of fact, it's not about the orgasm at all. Why not?

> **Orgasm:**
> Anything happening in your genital region that includes contraction, energy rushes, and pure joy in the body. Ejaculation is not a necessary component of orgasm, but it is most often present.

Because after the orgasm, it's over. The fun and games are gone, and everybody calms down. That's the point you want to put off! You don't want it to be over; so all the exercises that you've been doing with the 28 minute touch training and K + K and slowing yourself down and getting the rhythm of your breathing coordinated — that is all practice for this ritual. Because if you've got your body under your own control, you don't have to rush towards orgasm.

> **Climax:**
> The height of sexual ecstasy. This differs from orgasm in that one climax may contain several orgasms, but one orgasm is not necessarily the climax of the sexual act.

The rush toward orgasm is part of the animal self. We don't have to hurry up with sex before the giant bear comes back to the cave. We don't have to reproduce under stressful circumstances anymore; as a species, we're beyond that. We have homes so there are no threats anymore. We can hang out, take our time, and really go beyond just that carnal instinct to be over and done with it. Just as we have overcome our animal instinct to eat with our hands and crap in the woods, we can learn to have sex in a civilized fashion as well.

YabYum position

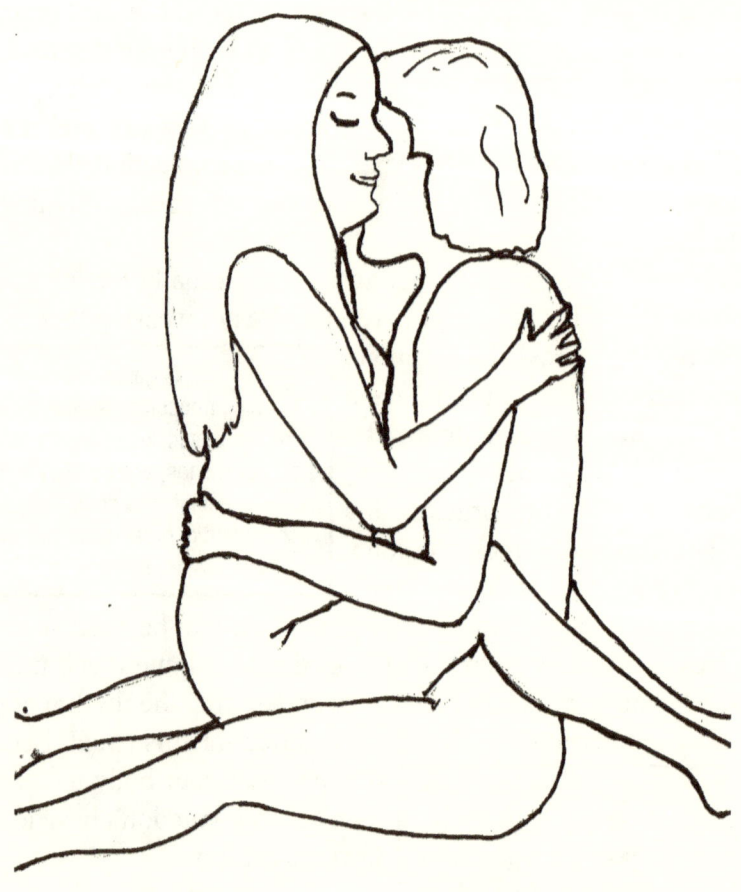

Yab Yum position has Shakti on Top

When you first started working with Kundalini I said don't cross your legs, don't cross your limbs. When you get into YabYum, remember that. You can cross your partner's limbs, but you can't cross your own. Kundalini energy will loop back around if you cross your legs, instead of going up (or down) and into your partner.

There are a couple of different positions that work very well for long-term coupling; YabYum is only the first. While it's good for learning, it's not the best one if you're going to be in that position for 3 hours. (See illustration)

It helps usually to have one butt up higher than the other, so you'll need a pillow. In a nutshell, the female gets into the male's lap with her legs stretched out behind him. She should have the pillow under her butt so her weight is not on his thighs. This position lines up all the chakras, even if there's a height difference. (Usually the height difference between two individuals is in the legs.) You also have your palm chakras, which can connect at the shoulder or anywhere along the route to the arm, which goes right into heart chakra.

The other thing about this position is that it's easy to keep your eyes on your partner's eyes. Begin circulating and breathing, sitting straight up. You can see it would get uncomfortable without practice.

The other position that works really well is lying down. I know this position has a name, but I've never heard it spoken. If the male is laying down on his side, the female can lie on her back and throw one leg over his hips and the other between his knees. It doesn't seem that everything lines up, but direct line up is not necessary once you have a solid chakra connection through puja with your partner.

(See illustration)

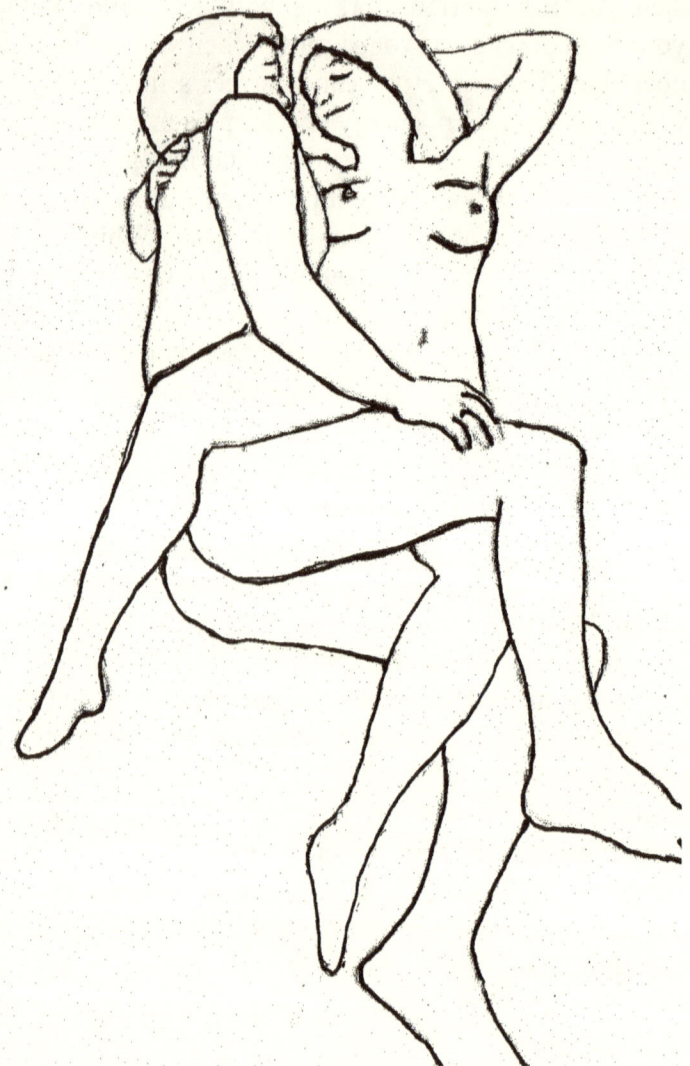

Position: laying sideways

    The Kama Sutra books have fantastic positioning and techniques that go beyond the scope of this book. As long as your ability to connect is still relatively sound, you can even stand on your head! No matter which position you use, the way that the chakras connect can help clue Tantric practitioners into more work that can/should/ will be done.

Maithuna from the inside:

Inside the Tantric priest and priestess during Maithuna is a buildup of energy. It's going down the male spine and up the female spine, becoming a cycle, turning like a turbine engine, or an electromagnetic generator. The couple begins generating energy, and once something is in motion it wants to stay in motion. The longer it cycles, the easier it gets to continue it.

The Tantric field forms around you. At the same time, the two people inside begin vibrating higher and higher. What happens to all of that energy? It draws itself together; it pulls itself gravitationally inward. There's this magnetism going on between the two people that they want to get closer and closer and closer. Since you're already about as close as you're going to get physically, with lingam inside yoni, the draw to get closer becomes the draw toward simultaneous orgasm. It becomes this balance between surrender and resistance. It's a trick to hold yourself between falling into orgasm and release, and keeping yourself from orgasm to gain more velocity in your energy.

Remember when you did the 28-minute exercise? Your energy built up in your body. Now you have two people doing that and running it together. It's going to keep building and building. As the vibrations get higher and higher, your consciousness starts going out of your body. You are hurled into trance mode, and you begin to get free flowing information that only comes through when you're in that headspace.

At this point, the two of you are blended: you're connected with the eyes, you're connected with the breath, you're connected physically, you're connected emotionally, all 7 levels are open and flowing. You lose the sense of individuality and the "I's" become "We." It becomes inseparable. You lose the ego, you lose the self, and you lose what it's like to be in your body.

Not being in your body anymore at the moment, or at least not aware of it as you normally are, the Naked Flame is free to do whatever it wants. In this high vibrational mode, we are not thinking technically or analytically. We are in the moment, simply experiencing. When we get into the Maithuna rite and really start running that energy, we lose time, we lose ourselves. Nothing seems to matter except to keep the ecstasy going.

I've heard it compared to the experience of psychedelic drugs. I have to agree that there is a very unique mindset that happens when you get into this meditation. You just keep going into trance mode, and it just keeps getting better and better until something happens. Usually orgasm.

This is why Tantrics, much more than ordinary healthy people, work so hard to be energetically clear. We practice disabling our habits, habits that we installed to stop or keep people out of our space. We need to be able to open up entirely, so when you get into this headspace and the energy starts flowing, it doesn't suddenly hit a negative spot within you or your partner. When that happens, one of the participants is liable to suddenly react negatively and jump backwards, or cultivate negativity over the next few weeks toward the other.

Some people have tried the Maithuna rite before their chakras were clear, and learned very quickly that it can be like peeing on an electric fence. They do burst into tears or find themselves very angry within an hour or two of the ritual. This makes some people shy away from doing it ever again -- or until they put more work into clearing themselves up. That's what I mean by a self-regulating system. The problem is not something keeping you from doing it; it's whether you have the skills to make it happen for yourself. Your own ability to be clear and your ability to run that much energy is the variable for this equation. You're generating that much more energy now, kicking in the Kundalini, doing all the connections, and something has to give. What give up are your consciousness, your emotions, and/or your ego.

Truly, in taking on this path, you're quite literally "asking for it." You're now putting Him and Her together, which are the creative energies of the universe. You're now generating a LOT of this energy. A lot of this energy. More than you can do by yourself. More than you probably have experienced ever in your life.

When you release that energy, you broadcast everything that is on your mind at that moment, and it creates the effect of changing your perspective all the way into your brain cells.

Tantra in the Brain

Intense energy affects our brains via a structure known as the amygdala in the brain. The amygdala's job is to regulate how we feel emotionally, and to react accordingly. Trauma of any sort will trigger it to set off a cascade of chemicals, which translate into signals, which result in an instantaneous and permanent change in the structure of your brain. This is what causes Post Traumatic Stress Disorder, or PTSD.

In Tantra, however, we utilize this natural property of our brain to do just the opposite; the intensity of a love-filled Tantric orgasm hits the amygdala as intensely as trauma does, but in a positive way. Under these circumstances, it programs our subconscious with whatever thought we hold at the moment of impact. What sort of changes do you think it would make to have a focus of perfect love and perfect trust between partners when that rush of chemical cascades hits the amygdala? It sorta blows your mind to think about how that would blow your mind.

Keep this science in mind when you practice. Realize that when we are generating this much energy it's really important that there's the intent of the highest good and love, and that there isn't an "oh shit" at the end of it. Especially if you went over the cliff into orgasm before you were ready. If, on the other hand, something silly distracted you, that silly energy could keep you from getting any serious work done. Make sure when you release that energy that you know where it went, where you put your attention, and that your focus was on the highest good, and not any hidden fears.

Be aware that every sexual act will create a bond between you and your partner. Without knowledge and control of chakra energies and your own reactions to them, you may find yourself immersed in more drama than you'd like. Accept this as the price of making love to that particular person, and deal with it by being honest, kind, and direct with all of the people you have sex with, even if 'direct' means 'goodbye.'

Exercise: Kundalini Connecting

This begins like the Tantric Field exercise, and requires a partner. Start with getting everything lined up and focusing on one eye, usually the right, for simplicity. Once you get into this, make sure your chakras are open. Take a moment, and focus on your base chakra, make sure that's open, second chakra, make sure that's open, third, fourth, all the way up. By now you should be pretty used to just sitting down and having them all open. Once you have all that going on, the next step is to open up your aura.

Visualize your aura like a big bubble around you, and open it to include the other person. Now you have two auras wrapped around two people who are gazing into each other's eyes, and have all their chakras open. Seal the chakras with an intentional touch or kiss. (This was in the Tantric Field exercise).

Once you are comfortable in this position, synchronize your breathing. As one partner breathes out, the other person breathes in. Keep an eye on the person's breathing. Breathe so that you can actually see what's going on. Breathe perceptibly, and of course, use Pranayama.

Now, as the Male or Shiva side breathes out, the energy should go into your nose, up and around past your third-eye and crown chakras, then down your spine and out thru your base chakra. As the Female or Shakti side breathes in, the energy should go up from the base chakra and out thru the nose. You will find that you can signal each other and speak while breathing out, which adds to the ability to communicate during this exercise.

You should feel a magnetism that wants you to pull you closer to the other person. Resist that urge. Stop and just try to hold still. Stop breathing for just a moment and see what the energy does. Does your body want to hold still? Not usually. Something in motion will tend to stay in motion. Return to the energy exchange, and continue to breathe in and out, getting the feel of moving energy between two willing people.

Recall the feeling of bringing Kundalini energy up in three breaths, and when both you and your partner are comfortable, begin to activate that energy and incorporate it into the circulation. You will find that both of your auras will draw down energy from above as one stream, and both will draw energy from below as one stream.

Now, using visualizations and internal focus, concentrate that flow into a smaller stream. Allow all of the energy to move, however, narrow the space in which it is moving to something the diameter of a pencil. This will concentrate the magnetism to your spinal channels, and reduce the amount of energy spread through your body, allowing the Kundalini energy flow to be at its most potent. You may find your bodies react to this as a shock; you may even find yourself leaping forward into the magnetism. If this flow is too intense, end the meditation and allow your bodies to adjust to the increase in energy in incremental steps.

Keep this meditation up as long as you can, and continue to raise the vibration until one or the other partner goes over the edge or backs down. To end the meditation, acknowledge physically with a nod or a word that you would like to separate. Stop the breathing and close your eyes. Embrace the person with a hug and recognize all of your energy as coming back to you and all your partner's energy as going back to them. Say to each other "What is yours is yours, what is mine is mine."

Then once those energies separate, back off from each other and ground. If you check your headspace, you may find yourself a little high. That's just the beginning. If you feel a little high from that exercise, you know you're doing it right. Experiment with putting distance between yourself and your partner and see what you can do with this new connection.

You can do all of this before and even without penetration. Penetration is the very last step, when the two energies can no longer resist each other. The reason it's the last step is that it's the bottom chakra on a physical level. You can't connect any of the other chakras so directly as you can that bottom one. Before you get into that penetrative situation, you want to make sure you can handle that level of energy intensity. Because once you're there, it's kind of hard to get un-there. If you're not ready, it's chaos on the loose. Some people do not survive the repercussions of this on the physical.

If you've done the Karezza and Kundalini exercise, ritual bathing, the puja, and the chakra sealing, then you should be able to continue resistance for a long time. Utilize resistance to put the moment of penetration off as long as possible. To build up the energy before insertion is a good way to insure lubrication. This way, when the resistance becomes too intense, the lingam can penetrate the yoni with minimal movements of the bodies.

If a couple practicing this method is not free to exchange fluids with one another, the female should apply the condom, and only when she is ready. This adds one more layer of resistance to the couple's ability to continue.

Speaking of Safe Sex:

White/Solo practitioners: If you have more than one partner within a year, you have some responsibilities that you must take into account with every lover. My students are usually adults, able to make the right choices in this department, and I'll treat the readers of this book the same way. You don't need the STD lecture here. However, I know plenty of people who, even in the 21st century, hate condoms. I would like to remind you all here that condoms are not the enemy--disease is.

Got a problem with "artificial" stuff being in the middle of your "natural" act? Then you should have problems also with the "artificial" cures your doctor will need to use to get you well again when you contract something. Seriously, if you have read this book this far, you are either ready to act on this information rather than react to contracting something deadly.

The solution to the problem of natural versus unnatural? Bless your condoms, make them sacred and hallowed so that when you touch one, the knowledge of this being a holy tool will change the way you feel about using condoms. (The same solution can apply to beds, sex toys, and intimate attire)

Exercise: Condom Blessing

Lay a packaged condom on the altar with the tip side facing down, and visualize Shiva energy coming down from above to fill the interior of the condom while Shakti energy comes up from below to coat the outside of the condom. Sprinkle their wrappers with water, and focus on the magickal properties you want them to hold. Place them in a cool dark place, wrapped in a natural fabric cloth, until you need them.

The other thing that helps is to set up an altar next to the bed, within reach during sex. Place your ready-to-use condom on the altar with the package pre-opened when you begin the ritual. This IS a sacred tool, more sacred than any other tool you've ever owned, and you should handle it accordingly. You can actually bless and make sacred any birth control method or sexual product you use in a similar fashion.

Getting there is half the battle

How many different types of meditation have we been talking about here? We've actually been discussing Maithuna all along, and all the things that are required to get to the point of being able to perform Maithuna. Maithuna includes everything we've learned throughout the entire book. Breathing, Chakras, 28-minute touch training, Balance training, connecting, finding The Inner Self in the heart cave, the Kundalini, the puja, the chakra sealing, and the sharing of Kundalini all lead to Maithuna. This is how you get to the state of enlightenment, which is the goal of Tantra.

We all know what happens to the body during sex. The lingam grows and the lining of the yoni gets thicker. The breathing changes, the skin gets more responsive. You have more fluids flowing in our genitals. The brain changes gears and focuses on the pleasure we are receiving. When you allow yourself to have full body stimulation, -- the whole nervous system orgasm as opposed to localized orgasm -- the chemistry in the brain creates long-term changes. Remember the amygdala? It is also responsible for releasing specific brain chemicals, such as the so-called "pleasure chemicals" dopamine and seratonin, when we have intense energy in our systems. These chemicals flood into the gaps between our brain cells while we are in this state of awareness.

What is the end result of all this extra chemistry? In a process known as "long-term potentiation," brain cells engulfed by these chemicals rearrange their components to accept more input. In some cases, it grows tiny new structures. It's the same process we use when we learn new facts, or create new memories. Once your brain has adjusted, the only way to undo the changes is to never access those thoughts again, and only over time will those newly created structures break down. If you continue to activate this headspace, however, you will gain the ability to push more and more energy through your nervous system, as your brain grows to accommodate it.

Practicing Maithuna and drawing it out for as long as you can, raising as much energy as you can, will cause your brain to produce it's chemical messengers for a longer period of time. This does have a psychedelic affect on the brain. Doors open in the mind, etc. When you do psychedelic drugs, it's an internal voyage. Maithuna is about the internal as well as the external. It creates no drain on the system like drugs do, because it's completely organic. It's also what our bodies and minds were built to do.

Elixir

If you read any of the ancient grimoire texts from old Europe,

> Elixir:
> The combined ejaculate of two people, male and female, who have a psychic, spiritual, or magickal connection to one another.

such as the Goetia and the keys of Solomon, they mention this mysterious substance called Elixir. This magickal, unattainable substance never has an explanation. However, it seems to be the only thing that makes these spells work. Well guess what: here's the secret. Elixir is the fluids left over when the couple is finished Maithuna (not necessarily as known by that name), which will have an energetic charge attached to them. It is a physical manifestation of that energy. That's why there's such a nice safety net over all that scary magickal stuff. Because nobody can make it work without this secret.

These fluids have a lot of fantastic properties, like being able to hold a charge better than any other item, and being able to be dried, powdered, and burned or dissolved in water to release the energies. Whether male or female, you will have an excess of this fluid compared to what you find during ordinary sex.

I recommend being very careful with those substances. There's ancient Tantric texts that talk about ways to reabsorb these fluids, with certain tricks like drawing the fluids back up through the penis, taking the fluids in by mouth, and simply lying still linked together over night. The effects on the practitioners seem to be in the eye of the beholder.

However, if you're interested in more about the elixir, check the texts in the bibliography. I will say that nobody in his or her right mind would put in print every bit of information necessary for the elixir in one location. I have said enough here; you must discover the rest yourself.

The never-ending Orgasm

The end of Maithuna is not an orgasm in the typical sense of the word. It is something that you may have come close to while doing the 28 minute touch exercise by yourself, but it's much more intense than that, because now there are two of you doing it. It may even be the most intense mental emotional physical state that your body can intentionally get into. It's not like an ordinary orgasm. There are no words in English to describe it.

You'll know it when you get there....

One thing that happens for men as well as women is that the orgasm itself continues for many minutes, wave after wave of it. Women can have multiple orgasms wherein they keep getting off for 20 or 30 minutes. This happens to some guys too, in this situation. Although we hear about this happening to women quite a bit, a guy can also get into the state where his neurons are rushing with that same orgasmic energy for half an hour, 45 minutes, even up to an hour.

"Should I be worried?"
My co-teacher once got a phone call from a female student saying, "It's been like two hours, and I'm still getting off! I can't stop this orgasm!" The student had been having sex utilizing these concepts with her partner, and became worried when the orgasm wouldn't stop even after the sex was through. They had gotten out of bed, put their clothes on, and tried to have a normal day, but her body wasn't being normal. She said, "This is very strange... should

I be worried about this?" My co-teacher asked, "How does it feel? Is it good, is it bad?" She replied, "No, I'm enjoying myself." His answer was, "Well, continue enjoying yourself, and if it should persist throughout the next day, maybe call me and I'll come ground you out." Of course, the effect eventually dissipated without any help.

If this should happen to you, go find a way to ground the energy out, either through the earlier exercises, or through strenuous physical movement. Eventually, you will find that it stops on it's own if left without grounding.

Polyamory vs. Monogamy:

Many Tantric couples give their partners freedom to be sexual with others outside of the relationship. Other couples find that monogamy has a more desirous effect on Tantric energies.

Polyamory, or the practice of having many lovers, has its benefits as well as its problems. One benefit is that a Tantric who has many different lovers will have as many different experiences with reactions to the energies. This experience teaches a lot while also being quite fun. Another reason for polyamory is to learn how to love on many different levels, not just sexually; one student of mine says he has a different lover for each chakra!

Monogamy has its benefits as well. As they say, practice makes perfect, and practicing these exercises with the same person each time helps both partners learn it faster. The biggest benefit to monogamy, however, is also the biggest drawback to polyamory; the long-lasting, long-term benefits of a Tantric connection that exists even outside of the bedroom. Monogamy gives an opportunity for a circular energy flow to exist 24 hours a day, 7 days a week, without any leaks anywhere. Polyamory does not allow for the tightness of circuitry that monogamy gives us, and monogamy does not allow for the variety that polyamory gives us.

Often, classes ask us what happens with triads or four-somes in Tantric coupling. Is it possible to do Maithuna with three people? Honestly, the physics of the electrical work do not quite work out very well with odd numbers. One must have as many Shivas present as there are Shaktis. The reason for this is simple electrical physics, and the same reason that there are two plugs on a typical wall outlet; energy must have a circuit to function. So, while three people cannot do a Maithuna rite, four people could; another good reason to get creative in your Tantric work.

I highly recommend, however, that you not simply choose polyamory or monogamy and label yourself with it. There will be times in your life where monogamy works best, but there will also be times in your life for polyamory. If you rule one or the other out, you will be ignoring some of the best things Tantra has to offer in life. Let the Naked Flame decide how it wants to live in the moment.

Kink in Tantra:

Many students have found our classes via the BDSM community, and we have had numerous opportunity to see what happens when someone who beleives their sexual practices to be "kinky" learns the methodology of American Tantra. Surprisingly, many people are not aware that their BDSM activities hold a kernel of chakra work.

Opening up psychological barriers is a natural response for anyone practicing BDSM or in a kink relationship. Learning the chakras and the sources of those barriers is the key to taking that skill outside the bedroom. If you can let down your defenses while being a Dom or a Sub, you can do it anywhere.

People who feel sexy while dressing cross-gendered, or in all leather, lace, or latex will find that clearing chakras allows them to make sense of these feelings without the society-imposed guilt. Folks who are into anal sex, endorphin-rush sex, bondage, and other alternative activities will come to understand more about themselves and why they like these activities as they work these methods.

Can you perform Maithuna with bondage? Can you cross-dress and still invoke Shiva and Shakti? Can you circulate Kundalini via anal sex?

Of course you can! You can apply these methods to anything you are doing. Do your own experiments. You can come up with your own methods in American Tantra. That's the beauty of this path--it works on your individual psychology, without the inclusion of mythos from other sources.

One type of kink that does NOT work well with Tantra would

be role playing. (i.e. father-figures, slavery, babyhood, etc.) This is because being here and now eliminates that possibility all together. You cannot pretend to be something you're not while being focussed on your real partner in the present. Role playing during sex will run up against the "true, kind, necessary" philosophy, and you will lose the ability to move much energy between partners if they are role playing. You will find it to be frustratingly incongruent, and Tantric activities should be set aside for this sort of play.

Groundwork:

White: Catch up with all your other homework! You know which chakras need clearing, how far you can get with Kundalini, and where Karezza takes you. You should be able to bring up K + K energy in just a few breaths. If you can't do all of this, practice practice practice.

Red: Kundalini Connecting Exercise (described earlier)

Blue: Anything you want! You now have the knowledge to make an impact in your community. Use it! Create the community of loving caring people you've always wanted. Build the facilities and amenities your people want and need. Volunteer for those less fortunate. Get out there and share what you've learned. In this way, the whole world will be Blue.

Chapter 10: Parting Shots

I didn't write this book to become famous or rich on speaking gigs, but that would be nice. It's not about being the first to print a book called American Tantra, nor the first in my community to publish. It's about finding a system that will work to help people in any community be happy. It's about knowing shortcuts and tricks that will allow someone to heal and grow through whatever pain they have faced from having lived in American society. It's about helping humans become the best humans they can become, because I live among them.

America is about freedom, and so is Tantra. Freedom of the Inner Self to be the best it can be. Freedom from other people's ideas of who we should be. Freedom from the Power-over mentality that caused our forefathers to strike out away from their homelands in the first place.

Empirical evidence is one of the mainstays of American society, and this path offers only partially empirically supported data. However, just because we can't see the human aura, or we can't build a machine to detect it doesn't mean it doesn't exist. Absence of evidence is not evidence of absence. We just need to keep looking. And we will--Americans are tenacious, if nothing else.

This is a proven system that works, written by an American for Americans. It gives people a tool to heal themselves with; a tool that helps them be less worried and more empowered and happy. Whether it's a valid system for you, the reader, remains to be seen, however, the power is now in your hands.

Thank you for your time and energy.

Appendix A:　The Advanced Rituals

Woman's blood moon ritual

One of the most balancing rituals regarding menstruation and energy is this following Moon Ritual

Cast circle outdoors under a nearly New Moon during the bleeding days of your cycle. Wait for a warm month, and wear a long flowing skirt. Find a grassy spot during the day. Make plans to come back on the right night. Then sit down on it, removing all clothing (and sanitary products) between yoni and the Earth. Send grounding roots down from the base chakra into the earth. When you feel connected to the earth, visualize branches that reach to the moon. Even if you cannot see the moon, know that it is there and at its darkest. Pull this energy up from Base to Crown, utilizing your Kundalini skills to move it up. Make sure you have dropped some blood directly onto the earth while sitting there. (Doing the Kundalini exercise will most likely make your body do that.)

Meditate on the symbolism of returning to the earth part of what makes you female. This is recognition of Shakti and the energy she embodies within you. As you pull up more and more energy, be sure you are allowing that flow to go upward to the moon. If you feel you must, howl, chant, or sing at the moon. Fill yourself with the energy of the night. Allow your own inner voice to guide you on this one. I highly recommend this meditation for anyone who wants to bring forth the magick of the feminine.

For those who are physically masculine, do this meditation in a similar fashion, allowing whatever fluids you wish to replace the blood. I've known males to use wine, semen, and saliva in this meditation for Shakti. Get creative.

Men's Sun Surrender Rite:

My co-teacher and many other males I know recommend this rite. I've done it once or twice myself, and have found it to be more empowering than most women expect it to be.

Start with a sunny summer day. Find a secluded outdoor space where you can sit nude or barely clothed. Sitting with the bare skin of your butt on the actual earth, allow the sun to beat down on your head and shoulders for a moment while you begin pranayama breathing. Once you are comfortable, turn your hands, palms up, to the sun. On an in-breath, visualize the sun's rays becoming your Shiva energy, entering through your palms and your crown chakra. When you exhale, send that energy down your spine to the earth out your base chakra. With each breath bring in more and more sun energy, and run it through the Kundalini pathway, grounding it into the center of the earth, which is the corresponding Shakti.

When you feel you are empowered by the sun's energy, allow your muscles to melt and your body to slump over into a comfortable laying position, however that takes you. Feeling the heat of the sun melting you like candle wax, surrender all resistance in your muscles to the power of Shiva.

Meditate upon this phenomenon as you Will.

The Panchtattva Ritual:

Perform this ritual after you have been practicing this path for over 3 years. It is typically necessary when the student believes he/she cannot progress any further within the confines of his/her knowledge. It is "Initiatory" in the most direct meaning of the word. This ritual transcends the ego in a very intense manner. Its purpose is to make the practitioner very aware of the Self, and to be able to get rid of it. Do not take this rite lightly. Do not do this rite solitary--have at least one partner. It can include up to five people, including the person undergoing the initiation.

Again, this is a dangerous ritual, and I am only including it here for serious practitioners. I highly recommend it as a thought experiment or astral ritual first.

Begin with listing these 5 things:

1. A type of food the initiate would never eat.

2. Something he would never do to his appearance.

3. Something in which he takes the most pride.

4. The initiate's greatest fear.

5. Something that he/she would never do sexually.

Give this list to the Guides or the guru, who can design the rite to include all of the things mentioned above. This works best if the initiate has no details after this point. Obviously, some things you just can't do in a ritual setting, such as bungee jumping. If you cannot include something physically, do it astrally. (This is much less effective.)

Beginning a month before the rite, the initiate should be doing intense personal energy meditations, such as Kundalini awakening, Gnostic drumming, or ecstatic dancing, every day twenty five days. After that, the initiate should be doing NO energy work whatsoever for the remaining time until the rite. For the final 24 hours before the rite, the initiate should fast, drinking water only. During the entire month, the initiate should be celibate, which includes not masturbating. Don't forget that this rite can be dangerous, and if needed, use safe words to stop it at anytime.

Prepare 5 copies of a mandala of your choice (or your guide's choice.) Place them on all 4 walls of the temple and one on the floor in the middle of the room so that the initiate can see it. Also, in the middle of the room, prepare a pile of pillows and blanket to act as a 'nest'. The initiate should take a sacred bath, instructed to empty his bladder, and then sit in solitude in the temple space for one full hour. During this time, the guides prepare the food.

I suggest, especially since this rite tends to shock the initiate, to do this rite entirely skyclad. At the end of an hour, the guides enter the temple space, and perform a meditation to get everyone in harmony. This meditation should be somewhat long and designed to put all participants into a mellower state.

The first test, of course, is to eat the prepared food. The guide should present it as disgusting as possible. There should be some sort of awful alcohol served with it, such as Licorice Liquor or straight

Kailua, especially if this initiate is a tasteful drinker. The idea is to shock the sense of "this is what I like, this is what I hate."

The Second step is to change the looks of the initiate in a way that he/she will hate. Whether this is shaving off hair, bleaching or dying hair, getting a tattoo (if you can do this in temple, hooray!) or whatever, make sure that the initiate has an opportunity to watch it happen in a mirror. This is to prove to him that his looks are not his Self.

The third step is to have the guides verbally rip into the initiate regarding his pride. Insult him on a personal level, convince him that his accomplishments are not his sense of Self either. Do this with the initiate blindfolded. If the initiate is skyclad, the attack can be quite effective.

The fourth step is to make the initiate face his fears. The guides will have to work on this without the initiate around before the ritual takes place. Sometimes it takes blades and blindfolds, sometimes it takes bondage and humiliation. All of it depends on the answers to the first 5 questions. He must realize that his fears are not his Self, either. Moreover, the Guides should not be squeamish!

The fifth step, (this gets harder to pull off) put the initiate in a sexual situation he would never otherwise try. Make it as real as possible, and keep convincing him that his sexuality is not his sense of Self. If he breaks down emotionally BEFORE this point, he cannot finish the rite. If he releases his energy during this time in the form of orgasm, allow him to release and go to the seventh step. If he breaks down emotionally DURING this step, he may continue the rite. If he accepts this treatment without breaking down or releasing, go on to the 6th step.

Instruct the initiate to open his energy centers while laying face up on the floor. The Guides can paint any symbols or sigils that represent the initiate's tradition on his skin at this time. All guides should pull up direct energy and send it into his open aura, filling his chakras and all the corners of his aura. This energy should be as close to Source as possible, flavored with nothing but Unconditional love. If the initiate is utilizing Tantric principles, one Shiva at the head, one Shakti at the feet should be enough. The idea here is to overwhelm the initiate with REAL vibrant energy.

Sixth step: The initiate repeats whatever energy raising technique he had been using during the previous week. The idea is to get the initiate to increase his energy to exploding point, and then dump every ounce of energy left in his system in one big bang.

The Seventh step begins when he releases all of the energy. If the initiate has not released after the 5th step, he MUST take this time to masturbate until orgasm is completed, and this orgasm must be an energy dumping. If he HAS released during the 5th step, then he should quickly release all the energy in his system in the most convenient way for him. His focus should be only on transcending this plane, and he should allow his mind to float as long and as far as possible. The guides may leave the room, and the initiate may wish to sleep in the temple.

The initiate will achieve a state of mind not possible any other way. This is initiatory, educational, and enlightening, and will likely change the state of the Initiate's mind forever after.

Appendix B: Modern Science meets Tantric Training

The problem:

Humans have been known to react to a particular phenomenon that no one can explain via today's science: Group Think and Mob Mentality. These reactions have proven to be one of the banes of our species.Everyone from school children to Wall Street traders to the Nazi's have shown the propensity for groupthink. Most of the ills we suffer as a society can be traced to people not being able to think for themselves.

Science today is still grasping at straws to explain this, with barely-valid hypothesis testing shooting arrows in the dark. My hypothesis is that Group Think and Mob Mentality are artifacts of the human aura created by the subconscious mind. However, the human aura has one major problem; it's not detectable by instruments that are scientifically "reliable." Perhaps because they are looking in the wrong place or wrong way for it. I intend to do everything I can to scientifically explain why and how people's energies can create such massive effects.

Where do "hunches" come from? What about intuition? How about psychic awareness, good guesses, and lucky streaks? If we can't prove the aura, can we empirically prove the effects?

I am open to competing theories on the nature of neurology, psychic abilities, and Tantra, however, without empirical evidence, neither side will ever win such competition. The race for empirical evidence that proves mental acuity and psychic awareness as we experience it is truly a researchable phenomenon is important for everyone on the planet. Indeed, it may be what saves us from extinction all together.

Consensus Reality:

Human beings have a problem in that they have to check in with "consensus reality" to function as a society. In other words, the question "did you see what I saw?" is a necessary function of society. This need for "consensus reality" has led every society to incorporate similar "unreal" concepts, such as ghosts and dragons. Either they accept or deny it, but either way, if at least one person didn't bother to say "did you see that?" we wouldn't have people talking about it. If ghosts or dragons didn't exist for all cultures at some point, we would not have a word for it in all languages.

When "did you see that?" is answered "No" by a margin greater than 1, that information goes back to the brain and we begin questioning our sensory capabilities. We take more time to scruitinize what information we get from our environment, and question our automatic inputs. With only a few repetitions, we teach our brain to disregard the most subtle of the inputs. By our second or third year of full-language usage, the we no longer believe that we are experiencing those subtle energies. After all, nobody else can see that ghost, right?

If the growing brain is convinced that there is no such energy to see, all possible routes of information flow are cut off so that growth energy can be directed to more used portions of the brain. This is why most people cannot see subtle energies unless they are "loud and in your face." They have to be able to affect other sensory pathways, such as the audio, smell, or kinestetic inputs, like the heat waves from a stove or hot asphault. If this energy is detectable, then aura energy can be detected as well.

The basis of intelligence.

If you're convinced that something doesn't exist, the brain will not allow you to see it. This is a little trick our brains play to keep our sanity. But, if you're already aware that something is what it truly looks to be, your eye accepts the details that are there.

This gives us a very logical theory as to why some brains are able to do things that science says isn't possible. Scientists are already convinced that they CAN'T see or feel aura energy, so they never will. In desperation, they fall back on the excuse of "future mystery to be solved." All they really have to do is forget everything they know, which is impossible for an intelligent creature.

The origins of intelligence is one of those scientific mysteries yet to be solved. Many have put forth conjectures and theories on how supposedly non-sentient organisms could possibly create sentience. One of the most interesting ones and perhaps one of the easiest to someday prove or disprove is the "Quantum Mind" theory, postulated by Dana Zohar, PhD. (see bibliography) Zohar proposes that it only takes communication between 2 cells to create a "thinking" organism, and that those 2 cells could be ANY 2 cells which are alive. (The definition of "alive", for the purposes of this sort of scientific endeavor, would be any organism that grows, eats, utilizes some sort of breathing, and reproduces.)

The second precept of Zohar's hypothesis is that when left to the second law of thermodynamics, all things that are vibrating will eventually be affected by the vibrations of all things around them as they gravitate toward entropy. This also involves planets getting stuck in gravitational orbit, piano strings resonating with a nearby instrument, and other observable phenomena. This theory has been proven more than once under strict scientific conditions. The most commonly illustrated experiement involves 100 pendulum clocks locked away in a room, set to swinging at different rates. Upon return to the room 24 hours later, most clocks are swinging identically. The logic behind this is simple if you think about it, but it's ironic in it's simplicity. Energy waves create wider waves which can then alter matter.

Let's say 2 single celled organisms are hanging out side by side one day, maybe in the air, maybe in the primordial ooze, and due to their proximity, their vibrations match. However, if the environment changes, and cell A picks up a vibration from the environment which changes how it was hanging out moments before (perhaps temperature or light). Cell B would –due Newtonian physics— necessarily have to change as well. This progression from Environment to Cell A to Cell B would be a very crude form of communication. It would be effective in the other direction, from B to A, as well.

Given enough time and repetition of this event, and given that things change according to their environment, it is quiet possible that these cells and their offspring would evolve to create a faster method of communication before too many generations had passed. As single celled critters evovled into multi celled critters, the benefit of knowing what is happening on the other side of the community of cells would be of such great evolutionary value, that higher and higher forms of internal communication would develop naturally.

What does this say about human behavior? What does this say about the cells in our body?

"Is there a scientific explanation of the chakras?"

The answer is yes.

There are 31 pairs of connecting nerve cells that run in chains down the outside of our spine, that are part of the Central Nervous System. These cells connect to other hubs, which are located conveniently in places where ancient spiritual traditions have located the chakras. While there are some chakra areas that contain more than one cell chain, there are no cell chains where there are no chakras.

This is how people with enhanced energy sensing abilities are able to pick up the energy of chakras from the surface of the aura. These chains of cells, due to their plural nature, radiate more energy than most other types of cells, and the energy they produce is also broadcast through the aura. This would be a good place to start scientific inquiry into the human aura.

The other neat thing about the human spine, which is a fairly recent discovery, is that some signals can come into the spine and exit the spine without ever passing up into the brain. This is how you are able to quickly yank your foot up from the ground faster than your brain knows you have stepped on something sharp.

These properties of the spinal column explain yet another aspect of why chakras function automatically, without much conscious thought. Try this experiment. Recall the last time you were ill to the point of vomiting. Think to the moment that your food actually revolted in your stomach. Now, check out what your body is doing as those thoughts cross your mind. If you're a fairly normal human, something funny is happening somewhere within your body merely by thinking about vomitting. There's a tightness somewhere as you think of it, probably the stomach area, but possibly also the throat.

That's your chakras doing their thing. That's also your neurons doing their thing. Your brain has created a thought pattern that is radiated through the body in a "body memory." These nerve cells create the energy that functions as our chakras.

The Crown & the Motor Strip

When you think about thinking, the mind is turning back on itself. If you try to visualize the inside of your skull at the crown of your head, in the same fashion, the brain is now turning back on itself. Tantra tells us that this crown point is important, as the seat of Shiva, the Lotus of Understanding. It is where the energy from above comes into our aura. Many people have reported experiencing a "shiver" down their spine when touched on that point unexpectedly. Many people have also reported that shiver when opening thier crown chakra.

What is at that point in the physical body that would give us that sensation of crown chakra opening? This is the point where two halves of the brain come together, left and right. Right below that point is the large band of connections that keep those two halves talking to each other. This is a very large, very central processing center.

Not only is that the point of division between left and right hemispheres, it's also the uppermost point of the row of brain cells that registers the sense of touch. Next to those brain-cells are more cells dedicated to movement of each muscle in the body. There's 2 whole maps of our body laid out in these two thin slices of brain tissue that runs from crown to ear on each side of our heads, one for sensation input and one for motor control output.

The crown chakra is where Left and Right come together, and also where the motor and sensory strips of the body meet. When we think about opening the crown chakra, our attention focuses on the central dividing ares of the brain naturally. Focus = more blood flow = more energy being utilized = more output of energy. Applied to the crown chakra, there's no wonder that crown chakra energy messes with people and makes them shiver! It's a body thing, again.

Psychic awareness:

I've explained so far the way a psychic nervous system works, but what, exactly IS it that we are perceiving with these extra senses?

What we are perceiving is a direct result of other people's energy. Some people put out more energy than others. They run with a relatively high metabolism, which puts out more energy per minute. They are the most energy-producing human units out there.

Some people habitually put extra focus on their thoughts (and therefore their energy). These folks get caught up in the "stupid loops" of negative self-talk, or over-use positive affirmations, and/or repeat songs and phrases in their heads repeatedly.

Those who put out large amounts of energy AND have that habit of extra focus are people who I consider to be psychically dangerous to others, especially when in negative moods. These are the people who tend to create what I call "hitch hikers" on their own auras, and who are apt to throw out psychic missles on others.

The funny thing about a hitch hiker is that once created, it doesn't want to go away. It will hop from host to host if possible, creating havoc for anyone and anything that it can, simply to feed off the negative energy that such havoc brings out of humans.

Sometimes hitchhikers are created by years and years of negative feedback loops; if Joe Schmoe thinks he's a loser, and he projects that energy, nobody will ever let him win, and therefore his belief will be affirmed. This creates the most potent of these hitchhikers, that then gain so much energy that they can weigh down their hosts. Many times it jumps from parent to child, and we see the phenomena of abuse patterns in families. Joe Schmoe loses his lousy job, goes home and beats his kids to make himself feel more important…and to make sure that hitchhiker gets fed. When old Joe dies, Joe Jr. is trained into just the same kind of negative feedback loop that keeps the hitchhiker alive.

As for ghosts, well, they do the same thing, only they are attached to spaces, not people. They do things to create fear in you so that they can feed off your fear as you pass through their realm. Yum. You be good breakfast, available for a simple "boo!"

Those of us with the right neural programming can see these suckers, and host of other related human stupidity, as solid objects to be aware of in our environment. Like other people see smoke and know not to get it in their eyes, we see this garbage and know not to get close to it....unless, of course, we're being dumb.

To be able to mess with this and not have it get "stuck" to you, there's only one trick. You have to vibrate higher than the crap energy you're dealing with. Easily done, if one has their health about them. Most people have some unhealty thought patterns somewhere in their behavior, and only by tackling those unhealthy patterns can we raise our vibrations for a duration of longer than one night.

Raising vibrations is what you need to do to level it off. One unhealthy thought pattern at a time needs to be dropped, until you can vibrate high enough to be the one in control of the energy in the room. Then you're safe to handle a hitch hiker, and just about anything else that comes your way.

Tantra is about raising vibrations. When we raise our vibrations, we are putting everything into line as it should be. Hitch hikers, bad days, and other people's crappy energy are no match for a trained Tantric.

Mellow out your unhealthy thoughts, mellow out your nerve patterns, and mellow out your energy. This in turn will mellow out your environment, and you may live happily ever after...

Final question:

Has it been 3 years since you first picked up this book?

If not, go back and read it again. If so, then recommend this book

to your lover. You'll be glad you did.

Glossary:

28 minutes: The time it takes for your brain to switch modes from Right brained thinking to left brained thinking or vice-versa. At the 28-minute mark, your brain is in a balanced mode of thinking.

Abyss: The dark place in the back of our minds where we keep all the things we don't want other people to know about us, or the things we don't want in our thoughts.

Blue Tantra: A new variety of Tantra that includes more than 2 people.

Celibacy: The act of not releasing any energy in a sexual fashion, including masturbation.

Chakra egg: A visualization that sets a stage that allows one to examine chakra issues.

Chakra tones: A meditation wherein the notes of the musical scale are associated with the chakras during intonation.

Chakra sealing: The process of connecting two people's chakras together so that they may exchange energy without any distractions.

Climax: The height of sexual ecstasy. This differs from orgasm in that one climax may contain several orgasms, but one orgasm is not necessarily the climax of the sexual act.

Connections: Psychic links that allow one person to be aware of the emotional mindset of another person without the usual clues of verbal or facial expression.

Contraction: A shudder or shiver that runs through your body that culminates in your genital muscles.

Deprivation: To keep yourself away from an item or substance.

Dzogchen: Skydancing. One traditional school of Tantra that has been popular in Europe and America.

Ejaculation: The fluids ejected from the body--both male and female--during sex. These fluids may be quite intense in scent, amount, or velocity.

Elixir: The combined ejaculate of two people, male and female, who have a psychic, spiritual, or magickal connection to one another

Enlightenment: The state of mind that is the goal of most spiritual pursuits. The concept of knowing all that must be known to transcend one's own karma.

Excess: Doing too much of something. The opposite of deprivation.

Experience: When capitalized, Experience is a mindset of paying attention to the here and now with all 5 of your senses.

Flower bud: A meditation that becomes a diagnostic tool for chakra blockages.

Heart cave: A meditation that becomes a diagnostic tool for chakra clearing.

Horizontal energy: Energy shared via the heart chakra and palm chakras. Usually this energy involves the sum total of what the two can be to each other.

Karezza: A meditation that involves self-stimulation and bodily control. This becomes a clearing tool for negative energy.

Kriya: Involuntary shivers and shakes in the nervous system that represent energy leaving the body.

Kundalini: A meditation based in breath and visualizations. This becomes a tool for chakra clearing.

Lingam: the Sanskrit word for Penis. Also is applied to any upright object that could be symbolically Shiva's penis.

Maithuna: The ceremony that involves worshipping the partner, invoking Shiva and Shakti, and having physical sexual coitus.

Masturbation: One handed sex.

Meditation: The act of focusing on one idea, excluding all else.

Om: The seed syllable of the universe. A sound to focus on in meditation.

Orgasm: Anything happening in your genital region that includes contraction, energy rushes, and pure joy in the body. Ejaculation is not a necessary component of orgasm, but it is most often present.

Pocket fantasy: A fantasy that you use regularly to get yourself into a more intense state of sexual arousal. The "pocket fantasy" works every time you need to use it.

Pranayama: Breathing exercise that translates literally into "Energy Breath."

Puja: A particular ritual done by two people as an introduction to higher Tantric rites. Puja usually includes compliments, honoring, and gifting.

Red Tantra: Tantric practice that includes combining energies of two people.

Resistance: An intentional stopping of the flow of energy, due to fear or desire. The opposite of Surrender

Shakti: the Feminine aspect of Divinity

Shiva: the Masculine aspect of Divinity

Skydancing: A school of Tantra, known in Sanskrit as "Dzog-Chen" Tantra. This term also applies to the feeling one gets when successful at Red Tantra. Orgasms can be so intense that it feels like one is "dancing in the sky."

Spontaneous arousal: When energy levels raise in the body due to unforeseen situations or unintentional practice.

Surrender: An intentional relaxation that allows any energy flow to continue on its intended course. Surrender is the opposite of Resistance.

Tantric fields: The energy that surrounds a person or a couple when practicing Tantra.

Tri-chotomy: The connection of Mind, Body, and Spirit.

Twilight language: Metaphor and double-entendres designed to mask and veil the true meaning of a phrase.

Vertical energy: A Tantric field that orients itself with the top and bottom chakras.

Vibration: The result of the energy in your system. Healthier people vibrate at a higher rate than unhealthy people do.

White Tantra: Tantra performed by one person.

Yab yum: A position that a couple takes when practicing Red Tantra. This position has one partner sitting in the lap of another.

Yoni: Sanskrit word for Female genitalia. Also can be applied to any body opening.

Bibliography

Allen, Marcus. Tantra for the West. CA: Whatever Publishing, 1981.

Anand, Margo. the Art of Sexual Magick. NY: GP Putnam, 1995.

Bandler, R. and Grinder, J. Frogs into Princes: Neuro Linguistic Programming. Real People Press, Boulder, CO, 1979.

Chia, Mantak The Healing Tao series, Aurora Press, Sante Fe, NM, 1984.

--Cultivating Female Sexual Energy

--Cultivating Male Sexual Energy

Crowley, Aleister. Magick in Theory and Practice. Edison, NJ: Castle, 1991.

Dahlke, Rudiger. Mandalas of the World: A Meditating and Painting Guide (Paperback) NY: Sterling 2004.

Deveney, John Patrick. Paschal Beverly Randolph, A Nineteenth Century Black American Spiritualist, Rosicrucian, and Sex Magician State University of New York Press, 1997.

Dowman, Keith. Skydancer; the Secret Life and Songs of Yeshe Tsogyle,RKP, London, 1983.

Firefox, LaSara. Sexy Witch. Woodbury, MN: Llewellyn, 2005.

Feuerstein, Georg. Tantra; the Path of Ecstasy. Boston: Shambalah, 1998.

Garrison, Omar. Tantra the Yoga of Sex, NY: Causeway, 1964.

Goldberg, B.Z. The Sacred Fire; the story of Sex in Religion, NY: Grove, 1958.

Hay, Louise L. You can heal your Life. Carlsbad, CA: Hay House, 2004.

Katz, Jackson. "Tough Guise". Los Angeles: Media Education Foundation video.

Kraig, Donald Michael. Modern Sex Magick. Woodbury, MN, Llewellyn, 2001.

Mumford, John. Ecstasy through Tantra. Woodbury, MN, Llewellyn

Murphy, Yolanda. Women of the Forest, Columbia Univeristy Press, 1974

Nema. Ma'at Magick York Beach, ME: Weiser, 1995.

Pinker, Steven. The language Instinct , NY: Harper Collins 1994.

Ramachandran, V.S., and Blakeslee, Sandra: Phantoms in the Brain: probing the mysteries of the human mind. NY: Quill, 1998.

Sinha, Indra Tantra the Cult of Ecstasy London: Nicholas, 2002.

Westheimer, Ruth K. and Lopater, Sanford. Human Sexuality, A Psychosocial Perspective. 2nd. Baltimore, MD: Lippincott, Williams, and Wilkins, 2005.

Williamson, Marianne. A Return To Love: Reflections on the Principles of A Course in Miracles, NY: Harper Collins, 1992.

Zohar, Danah. The Quantum Self: Human Nature and Consciousness Defined by the New Physics. NY: Quill, 1990.

Websites:

On Tantra:

http://www.globalideasbank.org/wbi/WBI-20.HTML

http://www.luckymojo.com/sacredsex.html

http://www.worldinter.net/~mstilwell/spirit/index.html

http://www.tantra.org

On Science:

www.bartleby.com/107/214.html---Human Anatomy

https://implicit.harvard.edu/implicit/---Implicit bias test.

http://serendip.brynmawr.edu/bb/neuro/neuro01/web1/Burdick. html. ---studies on PTSD.

http://www.lyricsdownload.com/acdc-the-jack-lyrics.html---Song Lyrics - AC/DC -- "The Jack" TNT (Aus) (1975), High Voltage (1976). Young, Young, and Scott.

www.ingramcontent.com/pod-product-compliance
Lightning Source LLC
Chambersburg PA
CBHW031320290526
45784CB00014B/413